# *Tim* NEALE

## MY LIFE OF

## ADVENTURE

# *Tim*NEALE

## MY LIFE OF

## ADVENTURE

An oral history of adventure, misadventure, and living

fully as told by Timothy F. Neale.

Audio recorded by Jesus Torres

Prepared and edited by Bonnie L. Campbell

# COPYRIGHT & PUBLICATION

Also available in large print (published in accord with the standards of N.A.V.H.) and EPUB formats.
ISBN: 978-1-941417-00-3 (large print), 978-1-941417-03-4 (EPUB)

Publisher: White Tern Press
Composition & Book Design: Bonnie L. Campbell, EnvisionNW Consulting, Inc.
ISBN: 978-1-941417-02-7
1. Biography 2. Alzheimers & Dementia 3. History, West (AK)
First Edition, First Printing 2017
Printed in the United States of America

WHITE TERN PRESS
SEATTLE

# DEDICATION

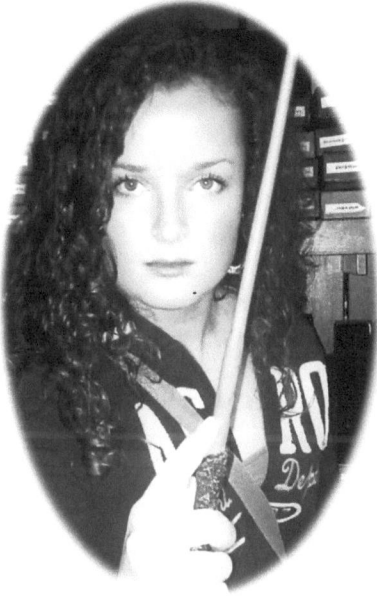

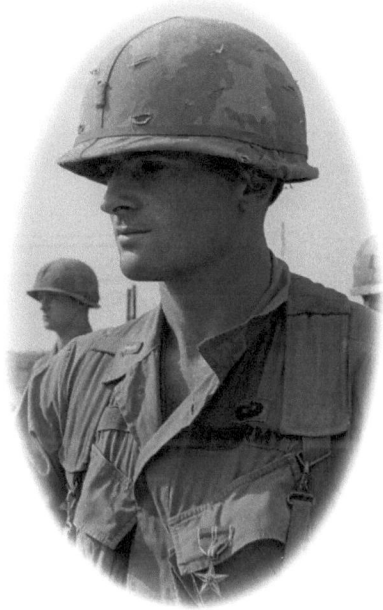

*I dedicate this book to my daughter Megan, and to those afflicted with Parkinson's disease. I am thankful that Megan has had the strength to weather the difficulties of this disease by my side.* — Tim Neale, Oct. 11, 2013

*It's not that I forget, I just don't remember...*

*— Tim Neale*

# CONTENTS

# ARTICLES & PHOTOGRAPHS

Thank you to those who generously have allowed use of their articles and photographs.

## *Articles*

## *Photos*

# FOREWORD

When I first learned that Tim was having difficulties, I wondered what I could do to help from afar. I have known Tim since the late 1980s. We shared several adventures as well as many stories over the years. Those who know Tim, know that he is a pioneer and adventurer as well as a story teller. It only made sense then, to begin this effort to capture his stories so that they could be shared for the future.

The stories have been edited to aid their flow (insertions noted in *colored italics*) and to remove some of the "ahhhs" and "umms," while at the same time retaining Tim's way of sharing his adventures. While perhaps not always grammatically correct, they certainly are interesting. Because Tim unfortunately has Parkinson's disease — quite likely as a result of his exposure to Agent Orange during the Vietnam War — the stories themselves are from his best recollections. So while some facts have been checked, it is wholly possible that they are not one hundred percent accurate. The mind is indeed a wonderful, yet fragile thing.

I personally am grateful for the opportunity to assist in sharing these stories. I'm also grateful to Tim's brother Roger, whose early encouragement made this effort possible. And also to our mutual friends who have continued to be supportive of Tim over the years, most especially now. Though it would be difficult to name them all for fear of missing someone, I'd like to specifically thank Liz Butera and Anne Leggett Billman who have shared in adventures as well as the more mundane tasks of helping Tim — working with and being part of his health care team as well as working with his legal team and the VA. Anne and Roger's assistance in finding and tracking down photographs was also most helpful. Tim's home assistant Jesus Torres (Jesse) provided critical coordination and assistance in obtaining photos from Tim's personal files while assisting Tim with his daily activities. I also appreciate the helpful eyes, understanding and encouragement of my partner Richard. Without you, this effort would likely be much more difficult, if not impossible.

With Jesse's assistance, Tim recorded the stories from his home in Anchorage, Alaska. Jesse forwarded these electronic files to me for bringing the stories together into, what I hope is a cohesive collection that shares a life of adventure and the character that I call friend—Tim Neale.

Let the stories begin!

*Bonnie L. Campbell*

# PREFACE

I would like to dedicate this book that I and several people have been working on. It will somewhat give me and other people a clue as to what my life was like prior to me having met these people. Especially my daughter, Megan Elizabeth.

I know that Megan has some apprehension about making a recording like this, she just doesn't want to see it as some big bravado trip just patting me on the back and her on the back. She just wants it to be real.

And I think that the book that we've, what we've done in the book is real. It's not about bragging about any one thing. But it's telling a story. And sometimes in a story you have to brag a little bit or you have to go out of your way a little bit to explain something. Otherwise it can be just meaningless.

I am duly impressed by the efforts that my fellow citizens, my good friends and folks have seen fit to take their time to work on relating to this book. A lot of them are curious about what I did forty, fifty years ago. People can also see the effort that is necessary to record what your parents and people were like prior to you arriving here. So I think *there is* some benefit in just using it as a guide.

I've had many people say—well not many, several—say "Hey, that's a good idea! You know, I was always going to do that, but I never got around to it." And that's pretty easy. 'Til you die and then that's the end of it.

# BEGINNINGS

## OUTDOORS
### Mount Spokane

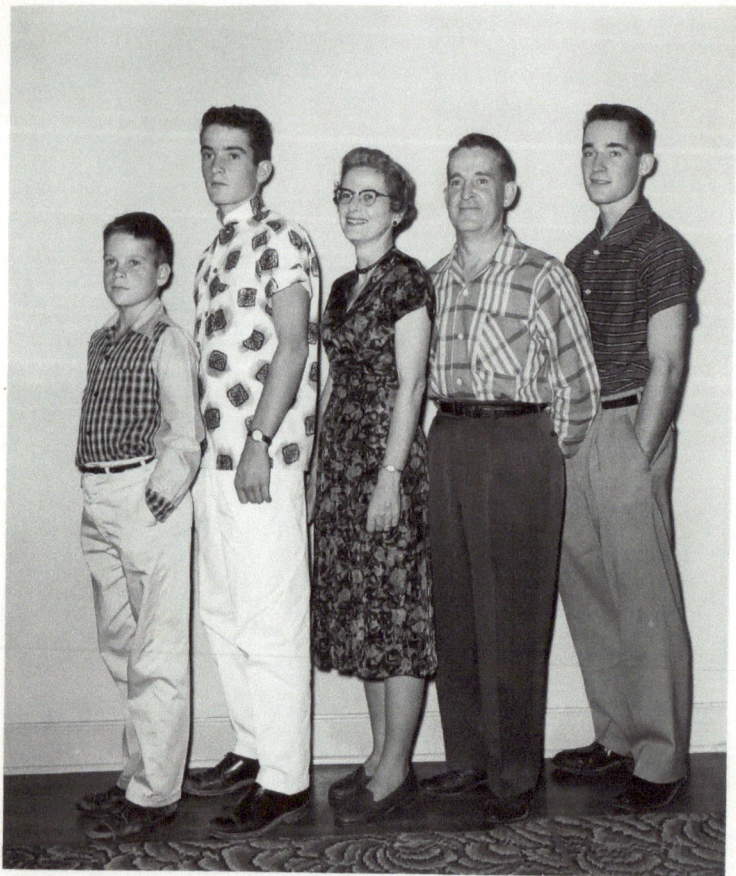

*The Robert and Goldie Neale family (Rick, Tim, Goldie, Robert, Roger), Oct. 1957*

Photo by Irene E. Dye

O f my many different trips that I have done through the years there is one that for some reason seems to slip my mind, probably because I never talk to anybody about it. It was a first really overnight hike/backpacking trip that I ever did. And I did it with a fellow cub-boy scout Rusty Kasberg. Rusty was a childhood friend. We lived across the alley from one another. We spend a lot of our summer times playing games and what not across the alley. Then somewhere along the line we decided — well, Rusty decided — he wanted to be a cub scout. We went on and he became a boy scout and I... not sure I ever became a boy scout. But Rusty and I did things. Like we'd go out on hikes and go look at birds and do various things.

One thing we did that I had to call him about. And I found him. He lives north of Spokane now in a little community. I had to find him and talk to him about this hike that we did many years ago. That hike was, maybe it was... the genesis of my desire to go out and hike and camp overnight and do things like that. I'm not sure where else I would have gotten the seed.

We were probably about nine or ten years old at the most. What we did is we got up one morning and my dad took Rusty and I down to the top of Mount Spokane. Our objective was to hike to Twin Lakes, Idaho — spend one day camping and hike the twenty miles or whatever it is to Twin Lakes.

Well it was kind of a mundane hike. We marched down through the ski area slopes. A lot of the area is either logged or mined. We got down about halfway to Twin Lakes that night. Camped that night, then got up the next morning and started hiking. Along the way we encountered two guys that were logging, cutting firewood. We chatted with them for a while and then we carried on our way. Early in the afternoon it began to cloud over. By middle to late afternoon it began to get really clouded over. And the next thing we knew we were in a thunder and lightning storm. Rusty and I decided the weather was getting pretty bad and we'd better get out of there. There's a lot of granite in this area — a lot of mineral — and a lot of reasons and opportunities for lightning to strike everywhere. So we started huffing it down.

We hadn't quite prepared for the rainstorm we got. We were soaking wet and kind of spooked by all the lightning and thunder. Pretty soon the two guys that were logging came tearing down off the mountain in their truck. They yelled at us to kick the logs off the back of the truck and hang on for life. Well, actually they said just to hang on. So we hung on and they drove like thunder. It was really, you know, lightning strikes here and there and everywhere. So we got off the mountain. They actually got us off the mountain and we got down to Twin Lakes much relieved.

There was a Methodist church camp that had some shelters built up on a lake[1]. When they saw us hiking along in the storm, they came out and told us that we could stay in one of the cabins and make a fire and get warm which we were very thankful for. But when I look back on it I think, *Geez our parents set us off on this little trip.* I still can't believe that my dad would take two young kids — nine or ten years old — up to the top of Mount Spokane (5800')... When I look back on it now, nine and ten year old kids just don't go out.

I wouldn't do this today. Or if I did it I'd probably do it with a gun. I wouldn't do it without a gun. You're just kind of naked out there in the wilderness. There are bear in there—in this area. Not a lot of them, but it would only take one bear. This is before I knew about bears. Those evil creatures.[2]

Anyway, that was my first real backpacking, hiking trip and it was a good adventure. I think that it was somewhat significant when I think about it. What on earth ever gave me that kind of a desire to go put my little backpack on my back and put my tent on the backpack, and gather up food for Rusty and I? Get our flashlight? Get all the little accoutrements we'd need for camping? And head off?

1    "Camp Twinlow," Twinlow Camping and Retreats, accessed June 26, 2013, http://www.twinlow.org. This was likely the United Methodist Church's retreat on Lower Twin Lake established in 1928. Their directions map shows the proximity of Mt. Spokane to Twin Lakes.

2    S.J. Komarnitsky, "Mauling deaths mark 1st no-sighting of bear that killed runners," *Anchorage Daily News*, April 17th, 2007. It's unclear exactly why Tim would call bears "evil creatures," but it may have to do with the untimely death of trail running friend Marcie Trent and her son Larry Waldron on McHugh Creek Trail in 1995.

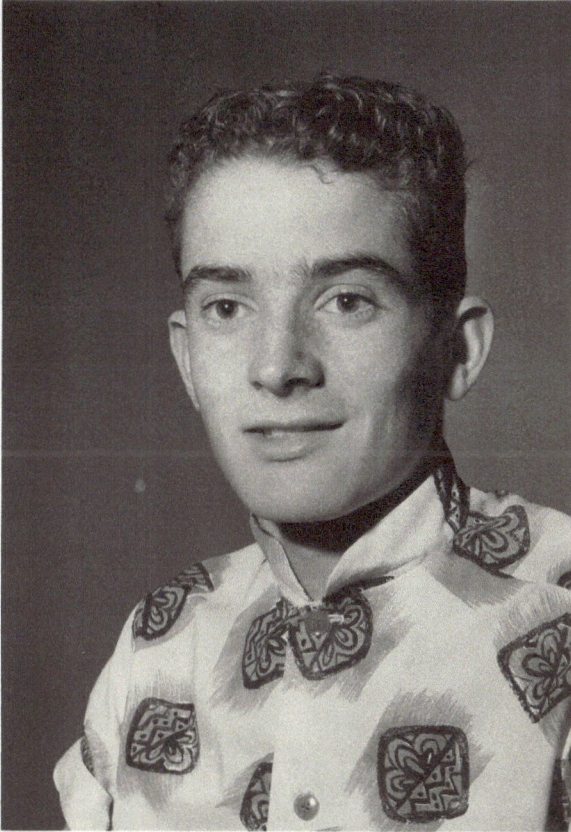

*Photo by Irene E. Dye*

*Tim Neale, Oct. 1957*

## Washington State Big Game Council

My real introduction to the outdoors, camping outdoors, building things out of doors was when I was selected by a group—an outdoor group—called the Washington State Big Game Council. They went around the state of Washington and selected a few boys that were interested in doing outdoor things, learning how to do them, and then camping out. At that time camping out was really just staying in a cabin. The cabin site was in the San Juan Islands on Orcas Island at an outdoor camp used by the boy scouts and girl scouts and outdoor groups like the one I was associated with. It was good. It was informative. It was a good bunch of people and we learned a lot. Things like how to shoot a bow and how to aim a rifle. I think also we shot some twenty-two rifles, but I can't be positive about that any more. That's many years ago. We also did canoe things. This went on for a month, I mean for a week.

When my parents showed up to pick me up to take me home back to Spokane, I was so exhausted I crawled into the back seat of the car and went to sleep. I slept about two or three days I think. Though they were a bunch of decent guys, as boys, everybody was still running around — visiting, trying to find the magic door to the girls and to the girls camp, which of course didn't exist. You take a bunch of boys and they're fourteen, fifteen, sixteen years old and it's hard telling what they're thinking. But I have an idea because I was right there with them.

I was very grateful to this outdoor group. I was never really clear on how I was selected except that my brother, my older brother, was the local president of this club, this organization. It was like a boy scout troop, and for some reason he couldn't go on this event at the last minute so the organization said "Well, you've got a brother that says he's interested in doing these different things..."

So I was selected and it was a bang up thing for me to do. I enjoyed it. Did have a lot of fun. It got me interested in the outdoors more than I was. Now I had an opportunity to do these outdoor things like the bow and arrow, the canoe. What else did we do? Playing with the compass, trying to figure that one out. That was a good one for all of us. It was a good thing and I had a lot of fun with it.

# SHEEP HERDING

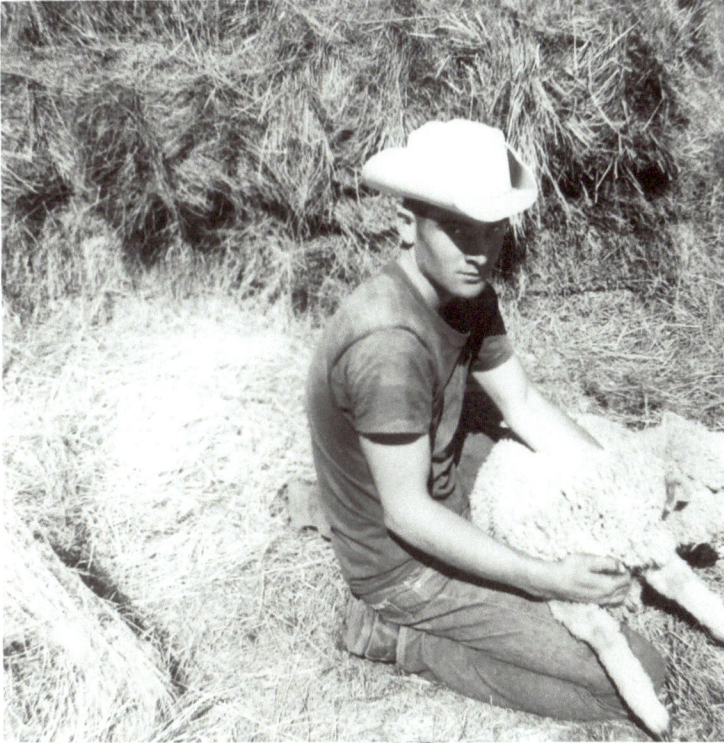

*Photo by Pat Milne*

*Sheep Herding in Montana*

## Ranch

I graduated from high school in 1960 from Shadle Park High School in Spokane, Washington. The summer before I graduated I worked as a lifeguard in a city swimming pool. The next summer I decided to do something a little more exciting and a little more daring. I had an offer to work on a sheep ranch in Montana.

My friend Pat Milne's uncle had a sheep ranch in Montana between Valier and Depuyer which is south of Browning. Pat and I, and a couple of other guys drove over to the ranch just to see it and talk to Jim, the owner about me working for him. He said "Fine. When you get out of school come on over and you can work for the summer."

Never having any experience working on a sheep ranch, I thought "this is going to be pretty exciting."

Anyway, I caught the train, the Northern Pacific, out of Spokane and went to Browning, Montana and got off the train there. Nobody knew I was coming. So, nobody was around to greet me.

*Wasn't I afraid to head out somewhere by myself?*

No. That didn't bother me. What was there to be afraid of? I knew I wouldn't get lost. But I did find out that there was something probably to be afraid of. After I ate dinner, I was wandering around the street and the sheriff came out and got me and asked me what I was doing. I told him and he said "Well, you know, this is an Indian town. It's not a good idea for a young white guy like you to be wandering around on the streets. Because, you know, some of these Indian boys are probably going to pick a fight with ya." So he said "I want you to stay in your hotel here, until I come and get ya. And don't leave the hotel until I get ya."

So I waited and the next morning he showed up and took me out to town where Jim the owner of the ranch was waiting for me to drive me down to his ranch.

Within about three or four days, I went from being a kid going to high school to a ranch hand on a sheep ranch with about 2500 sheep. We were in the process of getting ready to take the sheep north from Valier-Depuyer to the summer range which is up out of Browning or St. Mary's, Montana. I asked "How do we do this?"

Pat said "Well, there will be the sheepherder, me, Jim, and a couple dogs. And, basically we walk... following the sheep, guiding them along the way, trying to keep them on the road as much as possible. When we get to the bridges, try to get the sheep across them without getting them spooked and having them take off and run every which direction. And don't irritate the tourists—who want to drive down the highway and don't want to be stuck behind a bunch of sheep for a half hour—too much."

## Sheep Herder

Part of the time being a ranch hand was tending the sheep camp up in the mountains at St. Mary's, which is about one hundred miles from Valier-Depuyer. There your job became a camp tender.

You'd get groceries and supplies in town and then take them out to the sheep herder that was up on the range. He would tell you what to do and basically where to move the sheep wagon. Sheep could only be kept on one area or patch of pasture land for only four to five days. So every four to five days you would go up there to the sheep range and move the wagon and move the sheep.

Moving the wagon was an experience. I learned a lot about getting along with other people—like the sheep herder. He liked certain things. He always wanted his reading material from town. John J. O'Connor was about 80 years old and made his living being a sheep herder. If we were walking together some place, it was hard for me to keep up with this guy—and I was in pretty good shape! He just went in an amazing trot. But that's been his life.

Normally only one of us, either Jim or I, would go drive up to the sheep range and tend the camp. Some odd things happened.

One time there were actually three of us because Pat Milne came out and wanted to work a few weeks on the ranch. So we were moving the sheep and having trouble keeping them together because there was a bear or grizzly up in the area. It would get into the band of sheep at night. Well, actually it would get into them during the day sometimes too. But anyway, one night Pat and I took our sleeping bags and went up outside the wagon a little bit and put our tent, our sleeping bags and pad down on the ground and went to sleep. When we went to sleep there were 2500 sheep around us. When we woke up in the morning about 4 a.m., there was not one sheep. Something had spooked them and they took off. So the chore for that day was to get the sheep back together and get them where they were supposed to be.

You typically would go out and early in the morning with the sheep and you would get up and kind of guide them off the sheep bed where they slept at night. Then you'd come back to the wagon about 6 or 7 o'clock in the morning and you had time to do camp chores, make breakfast or lunch or whatever it would be. While the three of us had been up there, everybody drank coffee. Generally the way they made coffee is they had a pot that sat on the stove in the sheep herder's wagon. When you'd get up in the morning to make the coffee you'd just add water so you'd have a couple pints of coffee going all the time. The sheep herder had been grumbling because we had misplaced some of his stuff. One thing that somebody misplaced was the wash rag. So this gross thing was somewhere, supposed to be hanging on a hook and wasn't there. The sheep herder wanted to wash things up for some reason. He couldn't find the wash rag. About a day or two later, somebody stuck their hand in the coffee pot—and pulled out the wash rag. So this gross thing was in the bottom of the coffee pot that we'd been drinking out of for about four or five days—I thought it tasted funny.

## Sheep Wagon

It's hard to describe a sheep wagon. It's not big and it's got a canvas top. It looked like a Conestoga wagon. The back of it was a bed—just a couple planks and an old pad. So, if someone was in there sleeping—like the sheepherder, there wasn't much room unless you wanted to lay on the floor. Usually you slept outside. We never had a tent. If it was raining you could sleep under the sheep wagon. Or we might sleep under the truck or in the truck. But it didn't rain that much so it didn't matter.

### Parking the Wagon

Periodically you had to move this sheep wagon to a different campground for the sheep. When you moved the sheep wagon there was a certain way the sheep herder wanted it done. You had a door in the front and a door in the back. There were no side doors. So the sheep herder wanted you to park the wagon so that you had a cross breeze or had some air movement—especially if it was hot. It could get up to 60 or 70 degrees Fahrenheit, maybe even warmer than that. And if you had left his wagon perpendicular to the flow of the air or the wind or the breeze or whatever, it would be hotter than hell in there. He wouldn't be happy.

Another thing that would make the sheep herder very unhappy is if you drug his wagon up some place and didn't pay much attention to where you were parking it. If you parked the thing on uneven ground in such a way that he couldn't stay in bed, he'd roll out of bed. I didn't do it, but I knew who usually did it—who just drug the wagon up.

Sheep herders have been known to quit. But if they quit while there are sheep on the range and they don't provide for that, they can be ostracized probably for the rest of their lives. That could make life pretty miserable for the owner.

### Leveling the Wagon

How do you level the sheep wagon? Well, what the sheep herder would do—if he was up there when you happened to be towing the wagon around and he was close—he would come up and see what kind of a job you were doing. The way he figured out whether he liked the way you parked it or not was that he'd take his skillet and put a couple of tablespoons or so of water—put it in the skillet. And it was like a level. And if it all ran to one side, he wasn't happy.

So that is kind of the life of being a camp tender and a sheep cowboy. But from there we moved on to just the day-to-day routine of haying, bailing, farming. You got paid according to what kind of job you were doing. And if you were a normal ranch hand, you got paid $180 a month and room and board. By today's standards that wasn't much. By those standards back in 1960–61 it also wasn't much. But you were guaranteed a job and you were pretty much on your own. You'd get up in the morning and the owner would say "this is what I want done..." and then he'd leave—sometimes.

## Skunk

After bringing the sheep down or leaving the sheep range up at Browning. It's time to go back to the job of farming, plowing, seeding, and just taking care of the ranch. One of the things that had to be done was we had the summer fallow[3]—the crop that had been grown last year—and needed to get it tilled back up.

---

3    Blair McClinton, "Summerfallow," in the *Encyclopedia of Saskatchewan*. Regina: Canadian Plains Research Center, 2006, http://esask. uregina.ca/entry/ summerfallow.html. Summer fallow is a farming technique where a field is not used for a year. Typically this is done to raise the moisture

During this operation I saw a skunk—a momma skunk taking her babies across the summer fallowed field. And I thought *boy this could be cool!* I could get a little baby skunk, and take the baby skunk, make a pet out of it. But the only thing, the only problem is—how did you de-scent the skunk? And do you need to de-scent it?

It was pretty young, so I took the little baby skunk and put it in the gunny sack in the back of my tractor that held my food. He bounced around in there an hour or so until I got done working for the day. Then I went into the house to eat and told Jim the owner about the skunk and asked him if he knew how to de-scent it. And of course he did. He said, "Sure I can do that. So after dinner we'll take care of that."

So after dinner we went out there and he told me to go get the skunk. And so I held the skunk up by his tail—this little skunk was not much bigger than a baseball.

*Didn't I think that was a bad idea*—trying to de-scent the skunk? Well, it'd be a bad idea if it didn't work. But Jim seemed to think it would work. So anyway, I'm holding the skunk by the tail and Jim has his big bowie knife out there weaving it around and thinking that he's going to cut it. Well, he has had a lot of experience because he would castrate a lot of little lambs that were born and had to be castrated before you could ship them and raise them. So anyway Jim and I are sitting there and looking at this skunk and holding it up. And next thing we know this skunk can shoot a little spray—just kind of a little, looping little stream of scent and it landed on both of our clothes. So Jim just took the skunk by the tail, picked it up, and threw it out into the field. And that was the end of that—I thought.

When this skunk squirted on me, I had on a buckskin—actually an elk skin jacket. A real sturdy thing I used for hay—for stacking bales and stuff. But I was wearing that jacket when the skunk squirted us. So anyway about a week or so later, I'd forgotten about it and I went into Valier and went to get something out of the hotel. And I walked into the hotel and these old guys, retirement guys, were in the hotel sitting

---

content of the soil and allow the prior year's crop to decompose and return its nutrients back into the soil.

around there and pretty soon I hear this "Somethin' smells like skunk. Is there a skunk around here? What's that smell?"

Well, everybody knew damn good and well what it was. It was the smell of a skunk. And the other thing is, everybody knew damn good and well was that scent came from me — my clothes. And so the best idea I had then was just get out of that hotel. They weren't very happy about having that skunk smell so close to them.

So anyway I thought maybe that was the last I'd see the skunk. But...it wasn't.

Later that summer Pat Milne came out to the ranch to work for the rest of the summer. And when he got out there he'd picked up a six pack or half a case or anyway he bought some beer and so we sat in the bunkhouse and drank a few beers and laughed and giggled and what not. And I told Pat then that there was this skunk that was getting into the chicken coop and eating the eggs out of the nests.

And Cecile, Jim's wife, told me "You get that skunk outta here. I know that that skunk was the one that you and Jim tried to make a pet out of, but you get it out of here."

So I figured I well, might as well do that if the opportunity presented itself. Well, about two or three or four weeks — maybe later — Pat and I were sitting in the bunkhouse chatting and talking and having a beer or two. And then we hear this racket next door to the bunkhouse which was in the chicken coop. And I said "That's that skunk it's in that chicken coop again." I said "Cecile wants me to get it out of there, so let's see what we can do about getting it out of there."

So, I went in and got the shotgun. Jim had what they call an over and under shotgun, 12-gauge. So we went in the house, got the shotgun and brought it back out. And we looked around for the skunk. No sign of that skunk anywhere.

---

Often the fallow field is tilled to speed up the decomposition of the prior crop. The technique was considered a sound practice until the 1960s, but now is considered unsustainable due in part to erosion, organic matter depletion, and increases soil salinity.

Well, pretty soon I looked behind the door. When the door opens up it forms a crack, and nothing can get out of it because it becomes pretty narrow as the door is opened. And I look down and there was that skunk, looking up at me. So I stuck the shotgun — because it could fit in a narrow hole through the crack in the in the door jamb and I don't know what I was going to do with it. But anyway, what did happen was I inadvertently pulled both triggers on the shotgun and it made one hell of a noise. A shotgun by itself is noisy enough, but fire two of them exactly the same time — it's a lot more noise.

So, anyway, when I shot, when I pulled the trigger and shot the skunk there was total, dead silence. Didn't hear anybody from the farmhouse — Jim and Cecile. Didn't hear anybody out in the bunkhouse. Didn't hear the old herder. Didn't hear much of any noise and that lasted about — it seemed like about a minute, but probably just about ten or fifteen seconds. Total quiet.

And then, all of a sudden — there were about 50, about 30 chickens in that chicken coop –they all decided to come out of the chicken coop at the same time. And the next thing, Pat and I were still looking in there staying on the outside. Next thing Pat and I knew, we were covered with feathers and chicken shit. Chickens squawking, flying, clawing, clawing, trying to get out of there. And we thought that was pretty funny at the time, but probably wasn't funny at all. But, it made a mess.

So, obviously we never saw that skunk again. Probably wasn't enough of him left to even identify him.

Well, later that day we went in for breakfast, figuring that we were going to just catch all holy hell from Jim and Cecile either for shooting the shotgun in the building like that or else for making that much racket. Regardless, we never heard a word about it. And for the rest of the time I was on that ranch that summer Jim and Cecile never said a thing about it. And of course they had to have heard it.

# TIM & TED'S GRAND ADVENTURE

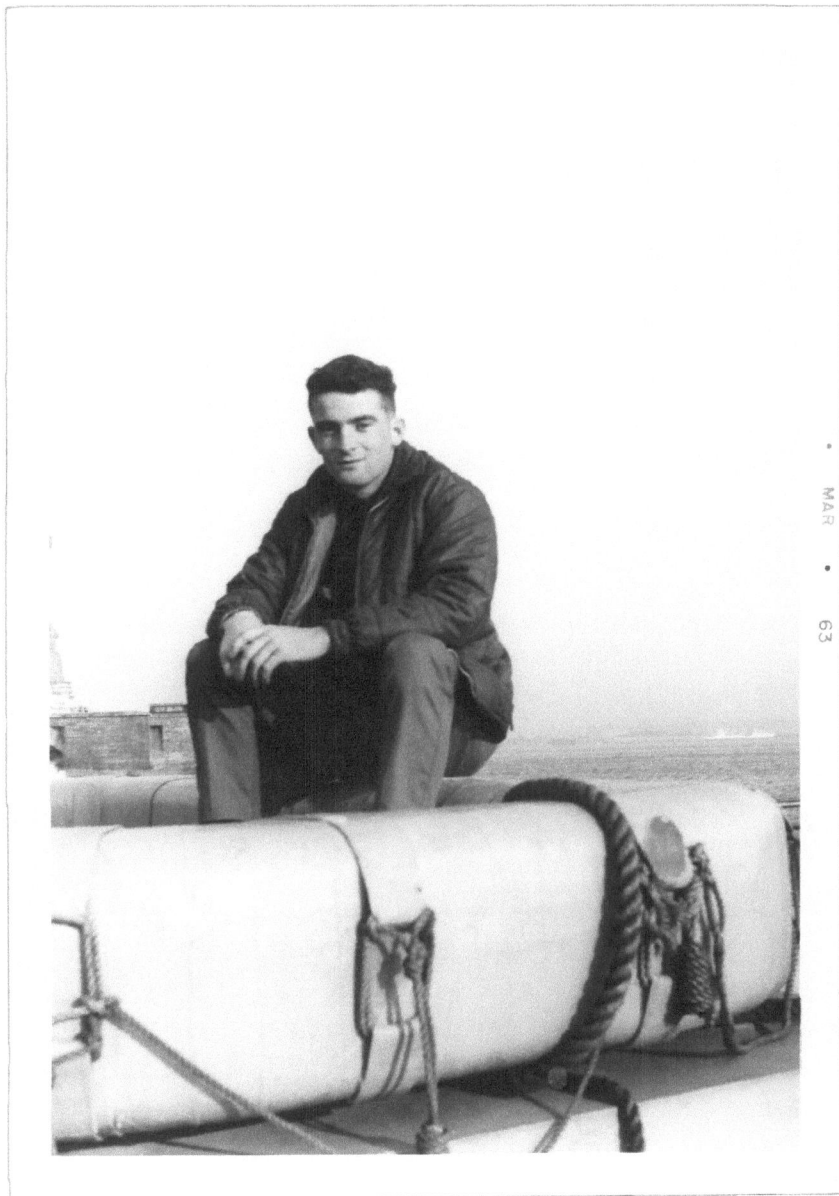

*Departing New York on the Osprey*

Ted Sheridan

## Europe!

A friend of mine—Ted—was an adventuresome soul. And one night we were at a party at Washington State talking about great ideas or great things we were going to do. But we had been that route before and hadn't really done much of anything.

So Ted said, "You know, let's commit ta going to Europe."

And I thought, this is a little ambitious. We were both about 18 years old. Thought yeah, I don't know about this but, he seemed pretty adamant about it so I said, "Sure I'll go with ya." And that's the last thing I heard about going to Europe for about a month.

Then Ted came back up to Washington State. We were at another party and he said "Well are ya gettin' ready to go to Europe?"

And I said "Uhhh well, well for what reason? Why? What, what, what am I going to do?"

And he said "Well remember about a month ago we decided to go to Europe."

And I thought—*geez we talked about it but we didn't exactly commit to it*. But Ted didn't think that, he thought we committed to it. And so I wasn't going to back down or leave him disappointed so we just decided Europe it was.

And so the next question was how are we going to do this? Well, I had an older brother that did go to Europe, and he went on the proverbial freighter. There used to be freighters going to Europe. Of course there still are, but you used to be able to work your way over to Europe on a freighter. And the way that worked was you'd go over and back and over somehow or another—end up being about three trips. But all that actually came to an end. And so, you couldn't ride the freighter over. However the freighters did have cabin space for about ten or twelve passengers, which turned out to be almost like a luxury ship. It had a stewardess and a steward assigned to the passengers. Of course there weren't any amenities on it, but they served the food. And it was all good food. You ate with the captain and that was a good deal. So how did Ted and I get into this?

Well, we hitchhiked to Europe, and left Spokane. And I'd been hitchhiking around the west coast quite a bit. And you usually got a ride. So I wasn't too worried about that. So we gathered up our bags and our suitcase and went down to the highway out of Spokane and hitchhiked and got our first ride. And that led to another ride. And I don't know how many rides we had, but what ended up happening is we got rides as far as eastern Montana. We hit there relatively easy hitchhiking. And then — no rides.

So we sat out one place, all night sitting there thumb out, trying to get a ride. And we couldn't do it. So finally, the next day we decided well we've got to do something. This isn't working very well. And it didn't work according to plan — whatever *that* was. So we got a ride into a little town, and the guy said "You can take the bus. It'll be through here sometime." We didn't know when. Didn't matter, we weren't going anywhere. So we got the bus and then that took us through another couple states and eventually we ended up out of Chicago. We didn't get a ride, so we sat around for a while, and pretty soon the cops came and got us.

And the cop asked us what we were doing and we told him we were hitchhiking across the United States. And he said, "Well, no you're not going to hitchhike across Illinois here. It's not safe and it's against the law. So what do you want me to do?"

The cop's asking *me* what I want to do. So anyway, we say "What can we do?"

And he said "Look. I'll do ya a favor. I'll take ya down to the highway, or this next town." I can't remember what it was. "And from there you can catch a bus and that will get you pretty close on your way. But you can't hitchhike on the interstates anymore."

So, Ted and I got to New York. And then the next thing we discovered was you just don't walk down the street in New York and get a hotel because they can be booked up or hard to find or whatever. But anyway, we ended up staying at the YMCA in New York, which aren't all that great accommodations. But at least we had a roof over our head. Then we had to decide how are we going to get to Europe?

And that was the next one that we decided we really blew. That was because we just assumed that there would be freighters going back and forth. We had heard that at that time freighters would sometimes take passengers. And the cost of taking these freighters is a lot less than like the Queen Mary or Queen Elizabeth. So, the next thing was, how do you get on a freighter?

So we went down to the dock, in New York and tried to inquire about passage to Europe. And where do you go? And how do you go about it? Well, finally some guy told us — what to do, and told us about an office that booked passengers mainly for freighters and they might be a good place to start. So, we hoofed it on up to this company that booked passage for you. Anyway, the guy said "Well, I don't have anything at the moment. But let me, let me just check. There might be a freighter comin' up that's got space, have two or three passengers that didn't show or somethin' and you might — they might put you on."

Well, it turned out they did. And we had about half a day's notice so we ran back to the YMCA and gathered up our belongings which consisted of couple shirts, couple shoes, and god knows what else and the old suitcase—didn't even have a backpack at that time.

Anyway, we found this booking office that booked these freighters. And went up to the office, and went in, and the guy said "Ya, I got passage. I've got a passage way for a couple people. If you want it, pay me now, because they're gonna go fast. Especially with a couple freighters that're just leaving now and have a tendency to take a few more passengers."

So, Ted didn't ask where the boat was going and I didn't ask the guy because I figured Ted had all the brains between the two of us. And I looked at him, and he didn't make any motions, he seemed to think that whatever we were doing was okay. So, we told the guy okay and wrote out our check. No, we didn't write out a check—we gave him our traveler's checks and took our stuff and went down to the boat, and I said "Ted, where is the boat going?"

And he said, "Well, don't you know?"

I said, "Well, I don't actually. My geography is not that good."

And Ted said "Well, you know, we better get a map." So we rushed down to an office that sold maps. Discovered we were going to Belgium. But it didn't matter to us really, as long as it was heading out across the ocean. We had initially decided to go to Northern Africa, but then we were advised before we bought the tickets, to not attempt to go to North Africa at this particular moment. So we didn't.

## Freighter

So after securing passage on this freighter that was going to sail in a couple of days we went down to see a few sights of New York and had just enough time to look around a little bit and get out to the ship. It was a Norwegian freighter called the Black Osprey and by freighter standards it wasn't a particularly big boat.

One thing that neither Ted nor I were sharp enough to figure out was that in March, April, end of March—somewhere in there, that wasn't exactly the time to be going across the Atlantic on a freighter or any boat. It gets rough. Winds blow. Storms come up.

And I believe it took us about six or seven days to cross. There were, there was cabin space for, I think it was six passengers. And it was a lot cheaper than going on an airplane. But as we found out later, it would have been a lot more comfortable for us if we had not taken a freighter over. We were in a continual state of almost seasickness and we didn't have any days of calm smooth sailing. But anyway, we survived it and got to where we were going, I think it was Belgium, and decided to start our trip from there. So from there we went down to Paris, France do some sightseeing and just to travel around.

We learned another thing. We had suitcases — the old kind that fold in the middle and you carry your clothes in. And periodically the suitcase comes open when you don't want it to and you spread your clothes and everything all over the ground. So we saw other backpackers and they had backpacks. And they told us, you know it's a lot more comfortable to be wearing a backpack and easier to carry, and easier this, and easier that. So, since we were in Paris, we found a store, a sporting goods store that sells backpacks. They were a frame pack, an aluminum frame pack, but actually a pretty nice little pack made of canvas— not like today's backpack. And not really secure so you had to be careful that things didn't dribble out of the pack accidently, because you used buckles and straps to tie the flaps on the pack.

So anyway we decided to dispose of the suitcases. And the only way we could figure out to dispose of them was in a garbage can or—I don't actually remember what we did with them—but we got rid of them and actually were much happier to use a backpack.

Well the next thing that we did, that we shouldn't have done, and didn't know enough about what we were doing when we did it was we decided it would be more convenient to get around on a bicycle. But we hadn't thought that one through. We bought the bicycles, got on them and started riding.

And the first thing we did is get into a traffic jam around the Eiffel Tower. They have this super set of roundabouts. It was like, twelve deep. And so you tried to get in one, and you try to get across, and the people don't give you any leeway and were honking at us. It was actually almost a terrifying trip, to get out there. And then we begin to have second thoughts if that was going to happen very often we wouldn't be better off with a bike.

So we foundered around for a couple days trying to ride the bike, trying to adjust to using a backpack that we hadn't ridden bikes with before. Up to that time I hadn't toured on any bike. All I did was ride on my bike around city parks when I was a kid. And we decided after some trial and error that the best thing to do would be take the bike out to a shipping company and ship it down to where we were going get on the—

Oh, that was another thing. We finally figured out how to get back to the United States. So we went down to book passage and this time the only thing we could find that was reasonable was, I believe it was the Queen Elizabeth, which was a luxury cruiser. A luxury line. They've got like an A, B, C, and D deck. So naturally we were on the D deck. And I swear that the shaft to drive the prop in that thing went right through our room. So we didn't get much sleep. But we still had to worry about these bicycles.

So to make a long story short, we didn't do anything with the bikes. We ended up leaving them at the freight company. Didn't recover them. Because, as we discovered, like a lot of other things we did without much forethought, it would end up costing more money to ship the bikes and getting them to where we wanted to go—needed to go. So, to make a long story short, again, we left the bikes there. Said goodbye to them and went down and started touring around. Then we could go to the different museums, and we'd go to Italy, Switzerland, and all these countries. And now we weren't encumbered with a bicycle or a suitcase. So then the trip began to get a little more enjoyable.

## Pickpocket

Well from Paris we headed down to the Mediterranean along the coast of Portugal. We discovered that it was actually very warm and great just to hang out on the beach and do a little partying at night, and sightseeing, and sleep most of the day. So the next thing that happened of any notoriety was that we decided to go down to Madrid to cash some traveler's checks. The way we traveled was with traveler's checks. You had to cash them at a bank or post office.

So we went down to the post office in Madrid and went inside and cashed our checks and I came outside and Ted was already outside and he was standing there looking at me. And I thought—*what's the matter Ted?* Seems to be a problem. He said, "That guy…" and he pointed at this guy who was taking off, getting ready to run. And he said, "He just pick pocketed me!"

And I said "What? We've got to get him, can't just lose your passport and your money." So I took off because I was a faster runner than Ted, and I figured I was probably as fast as this crook. But I caught up to the crook, and when I caught up to him I told him to give me back that billfold, and he wouldn't do it or something. And I banged him against the wall a couple times. He coughed up the passport. And the next thing that happened is I noticed these police coming towards me. And I figured, ah good, they'll take care of this bandit.

They kind of did, but they also took care of me. So, they hauled the bandit and I off to jail which was really just like a drunk tank. It had bars on it and a big, big room. And there were numerous folks in there sitting around doing nothing. And I looked around and figured out—this is probably not a good arrangement. And I don't know how Ted is going to get me out of here, but I hope I'm not staying in this thing overnight. And it didn't do me any good to try to talk to anybody, because nobody that I could talk to spoke any English. But somehow or other Ted got me released from jail. And I felt a lot better about that.

## Bullfight

We need the bull fight. So we decided to travel through Spain and go down and see a bullfight. The bullfight, can't say I've ever seen anything like that before, but there were about five or six matadors—I think—that came out and did their thing and fought the bull. And one matador was not quite as fortunate as the others. And it looked to us, Ted and I, sitting on the sidelines there like the bull gored the matador. And, not too much, I mean they pulled the guy off the bull's horns and ambulance people came out and took him away and the next day we found out that the matador was killed. And that's all the parts of the heroics of being a matador I guess.

So after the bullfight we needed something quiet, calm. We hitchhiked and took the train over to Portugal to the Mediterranean. Ended up hanging out on the beach for almost two weeks, just sunning ourselves and enjoying the times, the quiet times, and would go to the clubs in the evening and have a beer or two. We contemplated what next to do in our adventures here. We decided to go through Italy. And a lot of history. Go to Rome, Parthenon, Coliseum, and all these ancient places.

So we weren't going to go down into Greece. We decided to go to, go back into kind of, middle Europe. So we got a train to Munich, Germany and went through West Berlin. Actually East Berlin, and got up into East Berlin and spent a couple days there. Found out that we actually could go into West Berlin. So we took the opportunity to. They opened the gate, you know certain hours every day to go from West Berlin to or East Berlin into West Berlin is the way it went.[4]

---

4   Wikipedia s.v. "Checkpoint Charlie" accessed November 24, 2013, http://en.wikipedia.org/wiki/Checkpoint_Charlie. Checkpoint Charlie was the entrance into East Berlin from West Berlin during the Cold War. While the Berlin Wall was removed in November 1989, the checkpoint was not

So when we were in East Berlin we found out, we knew this ahead of time; that you had to get a pass. You had to get some paperwork of course to get back through checkpoint Charlie. So we were told where to go to get this. And all you had to do was to get a signature on a piece of paper basically. We had to go to this building to do that.

So we went to this building and gave them our paperwork and laid it down on the desk with our passport and this piece of paper. Then we sat down. And we sat, and we sat, and we sat. And I began to get impatient. I don't remember how long we sat, but it had to be an hour or two or three or four or something. It was a long time.

So I went up and I said something and I picked up my passport and Ted's passport. Actually it kind of looked like I slammed them down on the table this lady was working at. And that's probably the way it was too, but I didn't think it was very dramatic. And nothing happened. Then eventually some guy came and got us and pointed us towards the door and how to get back to checkpoint Charlie. So we got back to checkpoint Charlie and then we had to go through Checkpoint Charlie to go through West Berlin to get into East Berlin[5].

So when we went through the checkpoint, they detained me, I guess that's the way you might put it. And they asked me a bunch of questions and asked why did I give something to somebody in East Berlin. And I said I didn't give anything to anybody. There was about one or two guys that spoke some English, but they had me in a room and they got my attention. And I thought — *geez, not again.*

So after some interrogation, obviously I didn't have anything. Because I didn't. All I had was what was stuffed in my pack, which was nothing. And it took them about 30 seconds to look through that. And then they toyed with me and finally I had to take everything out of my passport and all my money. They wanted to see my American

---

removed until 1990. Tim and Ted actually would have crossed from West Berlin to East Berlin and back.

5    Wikipedia s.v. "Checkpoint Charlie." Actually Tim and Ted would travel through East Berlin to get to West Berlin. Tim was detained in East Berlin by East Berlin authorities.

money. Well I had taken an American $2 bill when we left the country and for some reason stuck that in my billfold, my passport book.

So in East Berlin, when they pulled out this $2 bill, for some reason the East Berlin authorities were kind of intrigued with this $2 bill. Probably because they hadn't seen one and, I probably lied about what it was for. They finally released me. And after going through this problem with Madrid and East Berlin, Ted was having no more of it and told me he would be highly po-ed if I ever got into any more trouble, Because the next time it could be they'd slam the door and –. And you don't mess with these people, the authorities in some of these countries. Take their job very seriously. Which is fine. So then we had to get out of East Berlin, go back over to Germany and go around Holland and Netherlands and any place else we wanted to go like that in Europe.

## Traveling by Train

Well, Ted and I discovered that probably the easiest way to get around Europe is on the train. One thing—the trains run all night. So you can hang out there and sleep on the train if you can. Then during the day you can site see and enjoy yourself. But anyway the trains are used by the locals too. That's how they get around. There's first class, second class, and we call it third class, but it's where all the people are that are traveling with their bags of groceries, bringing stuff in from the farms and what not. Since Ted and I would spend our days site seeing and wandering around, we'd be pretty wiped out and need sleep. And if we couldn't find a hotel room conveniently or whatever then we'd end up sleeping on the train.

The train had cars but there may be maybe four people, five people in a—you know what you want to call—like a room on the train. And there wasn't much room to stretch out. Well what Ted would do *when* he started getting tired and sleepy is he would get down and he would lie down in the aisle of the train car and sleep. He'd stretch out, but he was stretching out on the floor of the railcar. And that kind of impeded the ability of people to walk around. *Of course* this led to an annoyance by the other passengers, because Ted took the whole aisle up and the trains were crowded.

So the conductor would often come down when they figured out that Ted and I were together and of course Ted's laying here sleeping on the *floor*. He doesn't pay any attention to the conductor, so I'd have to go wake *him up* and say "Ted, get up! Get out of the middle of the floor." And he would say things to me that weren't printable.

But anyway, he would get his sleep and I would get chewed out. And in the morning I'd be tired, he'd be tired. We'd say "We're not going to keep doing this on the train. We'll get a hotel next night." But problem is, we'd get some place and there's no hotel around. So, we wanted to travel between two points so we get back on the train and get on this routine again of Ted sleeping on the railcar, me trying to fend off the conductor who was annoyed. And anyway traveling by train — that's how we did it.

## "Five Dollars a Day"

After we left Germany we were going to head for a visit to England, Ireland, or some countries like that. However I began to notice that Ted was beginning to wear out. He was showing signs of "it's time to go home." So I kind of had to go along with him and support him. So we decided, it was time to head home.

One of the problems we had is we didn't have a ticket home yet. So we thought we'd go down to the freight companies and see what they had. Then we'd go down to the big liners like Queen Elizabeth and Queen Mary and see what it cost to take a kind of a luxury liner to the U.S. Plus it was about half the time it took to get over on a freighter. So we ended up getting passage on the Queen Mary. And that was very luxurious compared to what we were used to, and it wasn't that much more expensive.

I have to say on this segment here that one thing we found very helpful at the time was a book by Arthur Frommer, called "Europe on 5 Dollars a Day."[6]

Well obviously, even then it got to be to the point that you weren't going to be able to do anything on five dollars a day. But the book

---

6    Arthur Frommer, *Europe on 5 Dollars a Day,* New York: Arthur Frommer, 1957.

was a good reference source. And it was helpful to us when we were going to be going into a place. Obviously we hadn't been there before and weren't familiar with it. So we'd get old Arthur Frommer's book out, look up the town or whatever we were and just see if we could get some names of just places to stay. Even though, as this book came out and was in circulation more and more people began to use the book. And most people who used the book were like us, looking for cheap accommodations, cheap transportation, and that type of thing. So it got to be — It was still good, but you couldn't depend on it being good for low income travelers. So it came time for Ted and I to depart. We checked out how much money we had and found that we had $80 on us, which was just the amount of money that the Greyhound bus lines charged to go from New York to Spokane. So I told Ted he could have the money; that I just needed $5 for food and I'd hitchhike back to Spokane from New York.

Well, on the boat I met these three people that were — actually they were Mormon missionaries. And they had just finished their mission which is a two year stint. And they said, "Yeah c'mon we're going to go to Cody, Wyoming" or someplace down there "we'll give you a ride that far."

At the time I thought "Well, that sounds pretty good."

## Cost

In searching through piles of stuff that I think are clutter, I found some journals that I had more or less done when I was traveling. I made one journal out of the trip to New York, well the trip to New York, but the trip to Europe. And I thought it was kind of interesting, because some of this stuff I completely forgot about. But just as a reminder, Ted and I did this trip on... Gee what was the date? 1964? 1963. So Ted and I weren't exactly what you'd call seasoned travelers or know the ins and outs of what we were going to find happen and I had said before, Ted and I were pretty naive. Because we thought we'd just go to New York and be able to hop a boat, go to Europe. And of course it didn't work out that easy.

But anyway, I don't remember the exact amount of money it cost me, but it was like $120 bucks or something like that; which on our budget that was a princely amount since we started off with probably $250 each. And that was going to take care of our food and lodging and what not for the next who knows how long. Well it turned out to be three months and I notice in this journal I got that we traveled pretty cheaply. Like a youth hostel in Paris was $2 each. And that included a room and food. Sometimes these prices would vary. We got down to Madrid Spain and went to a bull fight. That bull fight cost us 80 cents each. And we got into Munich and Berlin and places like that, it'd be more expensive. It'd be $2 a night. By today's standards that's nothing. But back then, I think it is relatively cheaper in those days than it is today with money exchange and all that. But in other words, it's probably a lot more expensive to travel today than it was when we traveled. When I took a bicycle trip around Holland, Scotland, Belgium and that was about ten years ago or fifteen years ago. It was about what it costs today. Expensive.

## Road Trip

Well, when I was about—let's see, 18 years old, maybe 19—my buddy Pat and I who were working on the ranch in Montana together decided we'd like to see some of the United States. And the way we decided we would do it rather than hitchhike, try to hitchhike, which can be hit and miss and you can get stuck in some places for 24 hours. And anyway we decided we'd take our earnings for working on the ranch and buy a car and use that as our transportation to see the world.

So we went to Spokane, because we had friends in the automobile business we got a pretty good deal on a, I think it was a '52 Chevrolet 4-door, good condition. As a matter of fact, the whole time we had that driving around I don't know how many miles we drove, couple thousand at least. We never had a breakdown, never had a flat tire.

But we needed to work periodically to make enough money to buy gas and food. So to do that we would just get jobs. This was in June I believe. July? April, May, somewhere in there. And we knew, since we'd worked on farms and ranches, we knew what needed to be done which isn't much especially if you're stacking bales. One job we had was in southern Idaho sacking potatoes which is a back busting job. But anyway paid pretty good while the potatoes were running. And then we actually picked up a few other oddball jobs. We'd go down to a casual labor office in a little town like Boise, Idaho or something like that. Get a job, lasts for two or three days.

As an example of one of these short term jobs, is we got a job installing seats that fold down in an auditorium, like in a movie theater. And you install these things, you had to bend over and put a screw on a bolt—a screw and a nut, and a washer or two on them. And after a day or two of bending over, screwing these things together, my fingers were shot, my back was shot, and I said to Pat "I'm ready to move."

So we packed up and headed on someplace else to sightsee. We went places like Death Valley. But it was so hot around there that we didn't hang around there for very many days. We went to Vegas and the Grand Canyon. Anything else that looked like it was a real touristy thing. But when you have unlimited time off and no purpose in life, for me anyway and for Pat, it became kind of boring. And there was no going out to throw the football around and play football down at the park with the boys.

So after, I think we were gone about a month or two, we decided it was time to pack it up, go home, sell the car. And get ready to play football that next fall. No, that's not true—we were out of school—we didn't play football. Anyway we just were ready to get back home and I was ready to get some job that paid me some money so I could go to college. And that was going to be Eastern Washington State College in Cheney. Gonzaga was, I went there for a semester or two, but it was too expensive for my budget. And I wasn't intending to go to law school which Gonzaga is famous for. So I worked the rest of the summer at a job building laminated wood beams which was worse than stacking bales but it paid pretty good money. So in the fall that's what I did until school started. And in those days you could wait until the day before school starts and sign up for school and get in. I can't remember how much it cost. It seems a figure like $350 dollars stuck in my mind. When I had been going to Montana State College a couple years before, I had a scholarship — a wrestling scholarship. And I was so smart in those days that I gave it up to go back on the road and knew that I could always fall back on the job working on the ranch. But that was a dead end way of living so I got into Eastern Washington and it was a good school. It was a commuter school for me and for a lot of students. I think there were four thousand students at Eastern in those days. And probably half of them commuted so it was a busy road. And you were always looking for people to commute with. Either you supply a car or they supply money to help pay for the gas.

So then I went out to the mailbox one day and I got this letter and I looked at it. And it was from the Department of the Army or whatever. And it said "Greetings. You are hereby ordered to report for duty." Well, I wasn't anxious to report for duty. So I went down to the draft board and I explained to them that I was back in school. They used to give student deferments. But they were beginning to get tight with those because they needed warm bodies on the lines in Vietnam. At the time I barely knew where Vietnam was on the globe. But anyway, that's a whole other story, being drafted. But I'll finish part of it here. They gave me a deferment for something like two months or something like that. So then I got another letter and this was a call up and they were giving me two weeks to put my life in order and report for duty. So that was I decided the way it was going to be and that was what I was going to do. Didn't necessarily agree with it or like it, but I would report for duty as expected as thousands of other guys my age were doing in those days.

# VIETNAM

## THE '60S

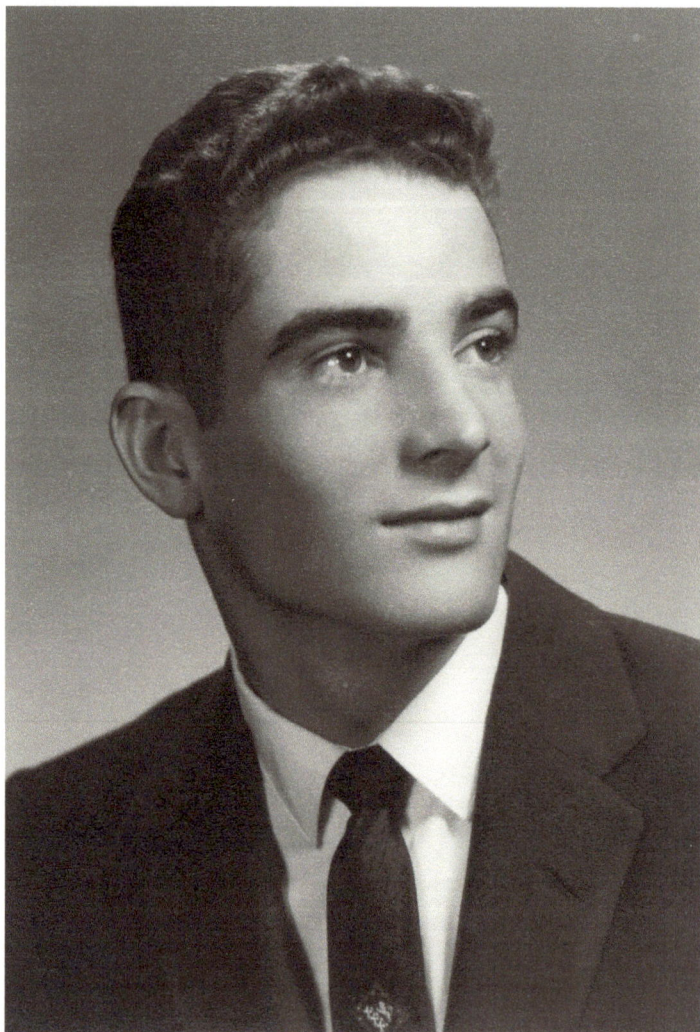

*Graduation in Spokane*

## A Path to Graduate

Well in the 1960s the war in Vietnam began to heat up and there was a great demand for troops, American troops. The way to get them was through a draft. So there were a couple things the military did. One was they wanted to get volunteers, try to keep an all-volunteer army. However that wasn't working too well, so they instituted a draft, which just plucked men off the street literally and put them in the army.

For me, I got my first draft notice and I went down to the draft board and told them I was in college and I would go into the army when I graduated college. Initially the draft board bought that. And then they came back and said "How long you going be before you go to college?" I told them a couple years and they said "Well, we'll give you about six months." So at the end of that period of time I was in the army. And there were a great number of men that had their lives disrupted with the draft. But anyway, they tried to make it about as fair as it could be. But the problem was there were a lot of guys that didn't want to go into the military. So they were allowed to be exempt. And once you were in the army, then you just became another soldier.

Well for me it finally got down to—like two weeks we've given you notice, you've got two weeks to gather up your stuff and report for duty. And I was sent to Fort Dix, New Jersey. I think it was Fort Dix. There were thousands of men just like me.

### No More Deferments

After high school, went to college, went to Eastern Washington and Gonzaga and Bozeman, Montana State College. At Montana State and Washington State I was on the wrestling team. But after I dropped out of school and didn't continue on my education, I dropped out of wrestling. I got back into college, but decided I needed to either do wrestling or focus on going to school and graduating.

When it came time to graduate from college, I was short one class, three hours of work, but I was short that to be able to graduate from college. So there was a lot of pressure to get that degree. I didn't want to go into the military which by then they'd already drafted me. And I got a deferment or two, but at that point in the draft world they didn't give out deferments anymore. So they told me, "About two weeks and you're going."

Well when it was coming down to the end, it looked like I was going to need one class that unfortunately was only offered in the fall quarter, and the fall quarter had already started. So what did happen is, my advisor, Dr. Elroy McDermott, said that what he would do is give me a directed study. In other words, I would go to his classroom and he would give me classwork for that one class every day or every couple days.

What this actually did, it gave me the path to graduate from college without going into the military and being three hours short. I didn't want to have that over my head, plus it would be hard to start back up studying, going to school, working. And it would be much better, which it was, to graduate and be done with it.

# U.S. ARMY

Photo courtesy Tim Neale

*Tim and his Jeep, Bien Hua, Vietnam*

## PLF!

After joining the army, I had several options available to me. At that time they needed helicopter pilots, and I thought well that would be neat. So I applied for the helicopters, but at that particular time in the military's career you had to pass a hearing test and an eye exam. And last year at college, my eyes dropped below 20/20 and I couldn't pass the hearing test. So I had to rethink what I wanted to do. And somebody said at the recruiting office "Since you're a college graduate, you can have the right to go to OCS — Officer Candidate School. And you can bypass a lot of the tests, get into the school." Normally it would take six months from the day you start till the day you get out.

So that's how that all got started. After I graduated from OCS, went to Fort Eustis, Virginia. And again I talked to the Army about becoming a helicopter pilot. And they said "Well, you can't make it, you can't pass the hearing." Same old thing. So I turned around and here was jump school. Airborne school. And I thought, well I'll try that. So they didn't care if I had bad ears or couldn't see. I was a warm body and they needed warm bodies. We found out later why there was such a rush to get people. And that was because Vietnam was really beginning to heat up. And they just needed people in the war effort.

So jump school it was. And that's an experience. Taught me how to stand in the door of a big airplane, flying along in perfectly good control and then you'd jump out of it. Well jump school becomes a real trip. One thing we do in more advanced training, just beyond jump school, they'll use two or four planes, these C-130s. And there are two of you in one plane and two in the other, and you'd alternate jumping out. Well, one of my experiences was I thought *"Who are these guys that pack these parachutes, and how often do they test them?"*

Well the way they do it—these guys that pack the parachutes have to jump out of an airplane using one or two of the parachutes that they have packed. So, that gives you an inkling of confidence I guess.

### Mass Jump

One of the other things that's a real trip, is when they do a mass jump. Like when they were going to do an assault with thousand men. And what they do there is get all these C-141s that carry, I can't remember, almost a hundred guys. And then you get ready to jump, and then the jump master will tell you to go. And when you go there's supposed to be a whole lot of other guys going too that are jumping out of this plane. Well, if you are in the front, it's kind of okay—*if* you're in one of the first planes. Because there's nothing in front of you. But if you're in the middle of this mass, it's hard to describe. But there can be, you know, a thousand paratroopers in the air. When you turn around and face them, these jets that they—including me—just jumped out of look like they're going to come and grind you up. So you want to get down to mother earth as fast as you can.

And the next thing that happens when you have all these guys jumping out at one time is the parachutes don't spread out. The jumpers don't spread out that much. So these guys are coming down. They land on your parachute. Then they land climbing over the edge of your chute.

So they jump. And then they teach you how to hang if your parachute collapse, you're supposed to hang onto the guy and ride it down with them. Of course the guy doesn't want you on his parachute because you're dumping air out of it. Basically you're not making friends with these guys if they're hanging on your parachute and you're trying to get rid of them. Or they're trying to get rid of you, by climbing up the parachute on the risers and dumping the air.

Then I went on to jump master school just to teach you how to — everything but pack the parachute. And it got time for us to do a night jump. Again they used C-130s, an ungodly amount of fuel. And there was — I believe there were either two or four of us — two on each side of the plane. And the jump master, the guy that controls when; he's pointing. You know. He points at you and, you know, you're supposed to jump. And then he points at the other guy. Doesn't take long to get through two of you, so of course you're not nervous or anything, you're just scared, the wits out of you.

So I got my turn this one night jump and jumped out of the airplane. And you can hear people on the ground, because you're only about less than two-thousand feet off the ground. And you can hear people and they're yelling at you. So anyway, this particular night, they were yelling at me and finally I could hear what they were saying. And they were yelling "Prepare to land! Prepare to land! Your parachute didn't open all the way!"

And I thought — *God, that's not good is it?* So, I got ready to do a parachute landing fall (PLF). And they teach you this PLF, to respond to a PLF with a parachute landing fall. You can be standing in the dinner line and the commander will come up and yell "Gimme a PLF!" And you just automatically, so you dropped and roll over on your side. And that's one time in my life where, well not one time, but one of the times when army training which seems to be redundant, was redundantly good to me, because I did a PLF. Of course my helmet came off in the process and it knocked me out. I didn't know what I was, where I was, or anything. And could hear when I finally came around, I could hear there was two or three more guys over me and they were saying "Is he dead? Is he dead?" And I was hoping they were talking about somebody else, but anyway we got that straightened out.

### The Box

When you jump out of an airplane one of the things you're going to need to do is to be able to carry your rifle, your bullets and whatever else you're going to need when you hit the ground. So they would have a box—a wooden box. They were actually old ammunition boxes, but anyway. You'd take this box which was about five-feet-high, five-feet-long and about a foot wide. You pack all this gear in it, then you tie this onto your pack—onto your parachute. So people who have parachuted, they know all this stuff. But just in case they don't I'll just point it out to you.

So when you wobble over to the door of the airplane, because this thing weighs about almost a hundred pounds. And it's awkward. And you need it with you. So you wobble over to the door where you're supposed to jump out. Well you don't jump with a hundred pound box between your legs. So when you hit the blast of air you say *"I'm dead, this isn't going to work."* But now the next thing to do is get rid of that box. So how do you get rid of that box? Well you can't just let it go and you're up there, you know, a thousand feet above the ground. If you let it go it's just going to be smashed to smithereens. So you have a cord tied to this box. And you release the cord. You should have it set up so you can release the cord as you're coming down. The next big trick is to release that box that is between your legs at a point where it's not going to start swinging and penduluming.

Well, in these big jumps, in where you're jumping a thousand guys at one time. There are guys that forget to tie their box on securely and so it comes down just like a bomb. And that gets kind of scary because again you know, there's so much stuff coming down in the sky anyway. Like guys lose their helmets and drop that. They drop the box. God knows what else is going to come out of there. But anyway, what you're supposed to do again is hanging in your parachute, and you look out on the horizon and when it looks kind of level out there—that means you can probably go ahead and release your box because there's going to be a point where you can't get rid of this thing.

So, it's a fiasco.

The army wisely decided in WWII, in the Vietnam War, dropping in airborne troops is not wise. It is not very effective, because for one thing you can't carry very much ammunition. I mean you have got a weight problem. And you know you can't carry a bunch of hand grenades and stuff that you may have trouble with later.

Well, there's a lot to learn when you're trying to be a paratrooper. The other thing is you've got to sometimes take vehicles with you when you go on a jump. Because when you land on the ground, then how are you going get around? So there were a couple things with that. One of them is that when you land on the ground in Vietnam you're probably going to be in the jungle or you're in a cleared area that we defoliated with our Agent Orange experience.

So back to falling out of the airplane. You get out of the airplane. The pack, your box is penduluming, and you know it's like swinging a ball back and forth at the end of a rope. And when it gets out to the end, your feet are sticking straight out and you can't do a PLF. Well, you can't do a PLF anyway, because of this box. You don't land on the ground and roll on your side. I never, I don't think I ever saw anybody do that and come out of that one in one piece.

Oh yeah, well here we are. We've landed on the ground. We've got some equipment. Howitzer and a couple jeeps with machine guns mounted on them and howitzers. So what happens is these things, these vehicles, are put on a plate or a platform and they're tied up so that when they hit the ground the parachute, the straps holding this plate on this platform, they're supposed to go sliding off. But that's another joke because a lot of times what ends up happening—because they made a mistake when they packed it—so in fact what happens is the front end may be held up and the tail end releases and everything gets smashed. Almost comical watching.

But one thing the army did do is they decided this nonsense of going into combat in using airborne troops and equipment is not very effective.

It didn't work in WWII and to my knowledge they only attempted one drop in Vietnam.

And it's kind of like, you go to the fair and at the fair there's a little pond with these ducks that are hooked to a chain and they go from one end of the pond to the other end. And you have this little BB rifle and you try to shoot the little ducks as they're going across. And the little ducks can't get out of the way of you. So you end up plinking them all down.

Well, that's kind of how airborne assault works. You're hanging up in the air. You don't sneak in there and do this, because—guess what? The enemy can hear your airplanes from miles away. Then you've got to somehow make sure you can see. If you land on the ground you've got to be able to see. So you need some lights. And that's another thing that doesn't help. You don't sneak up on anybody when you've got all these lights on and it just becomes something that the army hasn't repeated and probably never ever will.

## The New Unit

Well the next big event that happened in my life was going from Fort Benning, Georgia jump school to Da Nang in Vietnam. The army changed the unit designation of all the troops that went over with me from airborne to airmobile. In other words they went from jumping out of airplanes to rappelling out of helicopters, because it was a lot more efficient using helicopters than it was ground troops.

The army had to come up with a method of getting troops assigned to the 101st Airborne Division (Airmobile). So they went around getting troops from my unit, my company—a company is about a hundred and some people—so that I could operate and drive convoys up and down the roads. So they had to get bodies to do this—to drive trucks, running shotgun, and everything else. And the way they did this was they went around, and they had about a hundred companies in the 101st, and they went around to each company and said "We want you to give us one of your people to form this new unit."

Well, that had just a few problems. And one was—you can imagine what kind of people we would get in our units. Because if a company commander could get rid of any one guy by sending him to the new unit, which was me or us, then he would be rid of possibly the deadbeats in his company. So you can kind of somewhat read between the lines and imagine what kind of troopers they would get when they were assessing—it wasn't always the best person in the company. The company would send us, most of the time, one of the guys—who was a constant problem. But anyway, that's neither here nor there.

## Moving to Vietnam

Well after jump school, I was told to report to Fort Benning, Georgia and the decision had been made by the higher ups in the army to move an entire division of about 1500 men from Fort Eustis and Fort Benning to Vietnam, Bien Hoa. This was going to be a pretty massive effort. I went home on leave to see my family and what not. And I had to drive my car back to Fort Benning, Georgia. And when I got to Fort Benning, Georgia my company commander told me "Guess what? We're going to move to Vietnam, but this time we're going to go by airplane." So instead of loading up railcars in Fort Benning, Georgia and go through the Panama Canal on boats and railcars, we were going to fly.

So all of a sudden they started changing their horses, right out in the middle of the stream. And boy did that put pressure on our unit to move and get ready to move, now. My responsibility was to move the administration company among others, but the admin company is the one that did the payroll, did the medic work, did all the financing. So somehow the unit I was supposed to be moving had to keep functioning. The finance people, the medics, and all these people, they still had jobs. They couldn't just shut down for two or three weeks and move this massive unit over there.

So anyway, somehow or another, this was accomplished and the unit that I was in, we got to Vietnam and started getting set up to do the kind of a job we were supposed to do. And that was running convoys, moving supplies from the beaches to the supply points and the different camps. The different places like Bien Hua.

After the unit arrived in Vietnam, then life became just like a normal day night work job anywhere. Nothing exciting happened. We ran convoys. We'd run a convoy about every couple days. And most of the time the convoys were pretty mundane. And then monsoon season we'd be soaking wet all the time and when the sun came out we'd be cooking. And so you just kind of existed. Also you needed to wear what they call a flak jacket, which is like a vest that has plating in it so that if you got shot it may not go through the protective gear and you'd survive. But anyway.

# IN COUNTRY

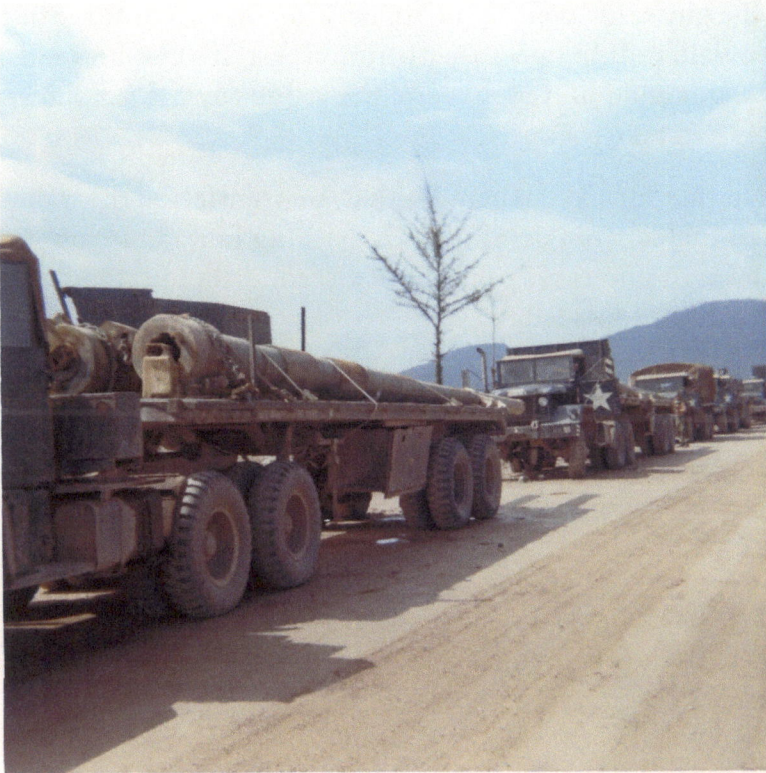

*Convoy to DaNang*

Photo courtesy Tim Neale

## Delivery

The day to day routine—just get the water for drinking water from out of the filtration pumps up to the camps. And that could have its problems because many times, not many times, but a few times I'd be out delivering water. We had these trailers that hauled 250 gallons and we'd take that water, set it out for these guys who were living out in the jungle. So that they would have a place to get—somewhat, you might call, fresh water—which turned out to be not quite fresh water.

But more than once I had the filtration people call me on the radio and ask me what I had done with the water that I hauled out of there earlier in the day or so. And I said "What do you mean, what did I do? I delivered it."

And the guy said "Well," — on an occasion or two or three or four. He'd say "Well, it didn't pass the filtration test. It's contaminated. So take that water and put it over there, where the guys have a shower set up. So they can take a shower."

So what that turned out being is that, we transferred the water that was contaminated from drinking it to bathing in it. So if you weren't affected by it in one case, you'd have a second shot at it. And we all found out what all this led to.

### Command Truck

Sometimes these convoys would last all day long. And you're driving on the highway — sometimes five miles an hour. And if you're not in the front of the convoy, you're in the back of the convoy. And the back of the convoy was not a desirable place because it was dusty. The other thing is — if you were in the back of the convoy, you'd have to be responsible for a couple wreckers. So if anything broke down, you'd hook it up to the wrecker or get somebody who was a halfway mechanic to repair it and keep it on the road and going. If we left the truck out on the highway the next day we'd come along and there wouldn't be anything left or else they would have stolen everything that was in the cargo. And that can be bad because we used to haul ammunition and howitzer rounds for the big guns.

The North Vietnamese in Vietnam were pretty industrious, ingenious people. And they were very intelligent. They'd figure out a way to wire up these bombs so that they become a land mine. When you'd drive over it on a truck they blow up. Well, fortunately for me, that didn't happen too many times.

We had formed up a convoy and had about three different units. In other words, three different army designated units and the marines. So we'd get protection for that particular convoy. It may be fifteen trucks long. And we'd have a kind of a shotgun effect with somebody riding with a howitzer on a jeep or machine gun. So if you were attacked you'd have some protection. On this one particular convoy, I finally had worked up in the pecking order to be the first truck in line on this particular day. And that was great. All my men thought that that was the best thing going because they would have much less dust and it happened to be a dry, dirty day. And they didn't want to be eating the dust of all of the other fifteen or twenty trucks ahead of them.

But when we got down to the marshaling area, and started lining up, these guys came over to me and said "You're going to be at the last today."

"What?" I said "I worked my way up to front and I get number one!"

And they said "We're pulling rank on you lieutenant."

And an officer of more rank, I believe he was in the marines, pulled rank on me and there was nothing I could do about it, except suck it up and not bitch too much about it. So down the road we go. And so we went from first to last. So here I am driving down the highway, and the land on either side of the road is swamp. If you get over there on the side of the road, you're probably going to get stuck. It would take a wrecker to get you out. And it would just delay the time that we would be out there and that my group would be out there on the highway.

Well, I can't remember how far we went. We went quite a bit of a ways down from the start of our convoy and all of a sudden there was an explosion. We looked up ahead of us. There had been a land mine placed in the road. And the Vietnamese wired it up to explode, which it did. And it blew the truck off the road. So I'm sure that the guys that were in that truck — it was a five ton cargo truck — they wanted that because they put sandbags, covered the floor with sandbags. They felt they'd get protection, but I never did exactly find out. I know there were several injuries, but I don't know how many were killed.

But if I had gone out first—I would have hit the land mine. They hit the first vehicle in line, because that's the one that has all these antennas. In those days we didn't have this high tech stuff, you had to use radios that had not much range, but had these antennas. So the command truck/vehicle usually had three or four antennas—whip antennas. And it wasn't hard to spot that truck/vehicle, five miles away.

So unfortunately at the expense of somebody else's lives, we lived because they put us at the back of the convoy, which I felt bad about.

But there's nothing good about war—nothing good about an experience like that.

## Thunk!

Well in a normal day we'd run the convoys up and down the highway. We've got somebody running shotgun on each vehicle. That person is responsible for responding if we were ambushed. Anyway on one of these hot, humid, or dry—I don't remember which way it was—days we were just driving down the highway about five miles an hour. Everybody—the three guys with me are kind of halfway fighting and dozing off. Some of them doze off. It's just so hard. There's nothing going on. And it's hot. They don't have an umbrella up over the jeep, over the cab.

My jeep driver is fighting the best he can to stay awake. The guy that's my machine gunner, that's sitting in the back of the jeep, is so sleepy he damn near falls out of the jeep. And me? I'm trying to stay awake. I'm supposed to know what the hell's going on here. But anyway, the three of us are there, driving along and we've got sandbags on the floor—a couple sandbags high. All of a sudden we hear this noise. And it was just a *thunk*. We looked at each other and then the three of us bailed out because we heard the noise and looked up.

Going across the dash of this jeep was a wire. And I had probably six or seven hand grenades hanging off this wire all the time. That *thunk* noise was the noise that a hand grenade makes when somebody throws it and it lands on the ground. So the three of us, when we heard this *thunk*, we instantly knew what happened. One of the grenades that was hanging of a wire on the front of the jeep had fallen onto the floor of the jeep.

Well we didn't know, but what happened was the detonator came unscrewed from the grenade, but it didn't allow for the spring to release and activate the detonator. It didn't activate the pin to hit the primer to blow the hand grenade up. So it was the big joke on us. When we dove out of the jeep, I'm sure it looked very comical to the guys following in the truck, which they had a big laugh about. We didn't think was quite so funny. Afterwards we had a great laugh about the whole thing. But that's after we got the truck fixed and back on the road.

So for the rest of the trip and probably a couple more, somebody was checking those hand grenades to make sure that we weren't going to repeat that and in fact have one of those drop down and have it activate the detonator and blow us up. And we didn't fall asleep.

## Ambush

It is possible you could get ambushed. We discovered that. And in the time I was over there we probably got ambushed three or four times. Gets kind of scary once in a while.

About a month or two or so after I arrived in Vietnam I was assigned a truck company. So I was running convoys up and down the highway. One particular night it was getting dark and there were only three or four trucks with me. We had cleaned up what we had shipped into the country, supplies whatever they are — ammunition for the big guns, barrels for the big guns, and just building materials for the tent platforms and whatnot. But anyway, we were coming down Highway 1 I guess it was. And we were to make a right turn and go about a mile or two up the road to where our camp was.

As soon as I made the turn, all hell broke loose. We came under fire and they — whoever it was — shot a rocket used to destroy tanks. It hit the flatbed truck that was in my group and blew up. Had the flatbed not been there, my jeep driver and machine gun guy who uses this machine gun when we need to shoot something *could have been hit*. I ran up the side of the truck to see what was going on. The guy who was riding shotgun with me helped. We pulled the one guy out of the truck. He was riding shotgun also. And he was in pretty bad shape.

So I ran back to my jeep and got on the radio and called for help. Told them we were being ambushed and needed some support. Well, it was right at dinner time and everybody was pretty laid back. Finally relief came and they were able to suppress the bad guys that were trying to wipe us off the face of the earth. Kind of scary. And that was about it for the ambush.

Sometimes people wonder what it's like to get shot at. And usually that kind of depends on how prepared you are. I was in the 101st Airborne Division and we spent a lot of our time training. And if you have good enough training you're taught to just react. So in this particular case with the ambush, we reacted. We got the machine gun that was on top of the jeep fired up and aimed in the general direction of where we thought the enemy was. But the enemy is beside the road and spread out in the jungle so they're hard to see. But you're being shot at. You hear bullets going and what not. And then if you lay down enough cover, and I liked to throw hand grenades. You could throw down enough to retaliate, then you may be able to suppress the enemy and yourself. Providing they don't have two hundred people in the ambush. But it was a welcome relief when my support people, men of the 101st probably just spit out their food, threw down their dinner, and high-tailed it down the highway to where I was. Or we were.

As a result of this ambush, I was awarded a bronze star with "V" device.[7] And hopefully we wouldn't encounter any more of those types of ambushes. However there were a few more incidences.

### Supply Point

Normally we went to a supply point to pick up our supplies. They came in on landing craft. And I'd take the trucks down there and load up our supplies and haul them back up to the camp. Well, for some reason, this particular time, they decided we wanted to go over to a different location and try that out. Different landing location because we had to be somewhere that the landing craft, the boats that we'd drive on and drive off, could get some firm footing so they wouldn't get bogged down or get stuck on the landing site. So anyway, this one particular day we went up to get the supplies and load up and turn around and come back and all hell broke loose.

### Dong Hoi

They had mined the road. And my counterpart, I think he lost a couple trucks in the initial ambush we had there. I didn't really have a job after the Viet Cong kind of circled in. And we couldn't really move

---

7    Department of the Army, "'V' device," *Army Regulation 600-8-22 Military Awards*, 6–5, Department of the Army, Washington DC, December 11, 2006. The "V" device is a miniature bronze letter "V" representing valor and is awarded with a medal to denote heroism. Each military/service specifies slightly different criteria for awarding the "V" device. In the Army the "V" device denotes heroism in combat with an armed enemy.

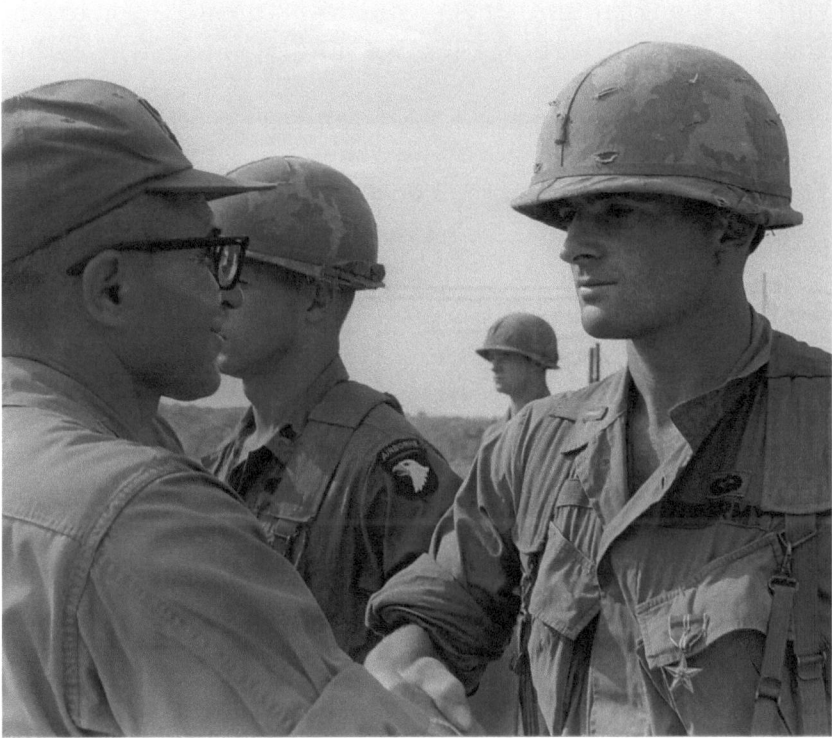

Photo courtesy Tim Neale

*Receiving the Bronze Star with "V" Device in Vietnam*

anywhere. We just stayed on this landing site. We had protection there, but there was nothing for us to do. Vietnam has beautiful beaches and one of the guys in my company was a Hawaiian. He asked me if we could go swimming. Well we pull our duty when we can, our guard duty, and then the rest of the time we just hang out in the tents because it's hot. So this guy asked me if we could get some plywood. So we went out and got some big sheets of plywood and cut them and made circles—something that was about 24 inches in diameter, maybe a little larger. And later in life as I went to Hawaii more often, I learned that what he had made us is now called a "boogie board." And if nobody knows what a "boogie board" is, next time you go to Hawaii go to Hanauma Bay—I think it's Hanauma Bay—and you can see them using boogie boards and body surfing.

So it seemed kind of odd to be in a combat zone and swimming in the ocean. It's probably about the safest place to be and not get hit. Only thing we really had to watch out was for the Portuguese Man-O-War.

These little octopus things that had stingers on them.[8] If you brush up against one of these little things, it's like running into a little barbwire fence or something.

So anyway, thanks to this guy's ingenuity, we made it a palatable stay. The Viet Cong had us pinned down, probably, I can't remember how long. It was three or four days anyway, before we could get back up on the highway and trudge on. But anyway, fun and games in Vietnam on the beach. One of these days probably when things settle down, Vietnam is going to be a resort town because of the beautiful beaches they have. And the scenery is really beautiful too.

### Defoliation

In this ambush that I spoke of a little bit earlier, ago I don't know if I mentioned it or not. But what happened in the next day or two the army would come in there with their equipment, their trucks with spray equipment on it, and spray the vegetation. Get rid of the vegetation by killing it all. They would spray where we were getting our water. So more than once or twice, I would send a truck, and we would go down and get water from a filtration plant that was set up. And I never got into it real deep, but there are no artesian wells or free flowing streams in Vietnam, especially out where we were at in the jungle. And I don't know what the army was thinking when they were spraying this stuff.

It was called Agent Orange,[9] which is like a form of DDT.[10] Very toxic. Well at that particular time we had, we were supposed to be taking a couple of pills. And one pill was a malaria pill to help keep you from getting malaria. But the pills were so powerful, that they

---

8    National Geographic, "Portuguese Man-of-War *Physalia physalis*" accessed November 13, 2013, http://animals.nationalgeographic.com/animals/invertebrates/portuguese-man-of-war/. The Portuguese Man-O-War is actually a colony of different organisms working together called a siphonophore. It floats on the water surface and is made up of a sail and tentacles that can produce a very painful sting.

9    Monsanto, "Agent Orange: Background on Monsanto's Involvement" accessed November 13, 2013, http://www.monsanto.com/newsviews/Pages/agent-orange-background-monsanto-involvement.aspx.

10    National Pesticide Information Center, "DDT (General Fact Sheet)," Oregon State University, Corvallis: December 1999.

nauseated me and about everybody else that took them. So you know we're just a bunch of nineteen, twenty year old kids. We decided we're not taking these pills. This stuff is, you know the pill was probably killing us more than the malaria would have. Now my life has been changed considerably by Agent Orange.

## Coordinates

During my stint in Vietnam for some reason I was under the enemies' eyesight or gun sights a few times. Get shot at. Putting mines in the road blowing it up, trying to blow us up. And just anything they could to try to blow up the convoy. I was running convoys up and down the highway. Anyway on one particular time, coming out of Da Nang and going up to Hue, we had a convoy and it was stretched out. The usual routine was I'd have maybe twenty trucks, ten, fifteen trucks stretched out—two and a half ton trucks, five ton cargo trucks. And we would be stretched out along a highway for several yards. We were supposed to try to get them to maintain a distant interval between vehicles so if something happens you've got some room to maneuver. But what usually happens is it ends up being bumper car a lot of times with guys right, one right on top of one another. I would run at the back of the convoy in my command vehicle, which had the radios and the antennas sticking out, so that if something happened I would be able to control it—hopefully—better than if I was at the front.

It was just another sleepy day of running the convoy through the villages. And we probably go, seems to me I remember, top speed would be probably twenty and more than likely we'd be going fifteen. It was just impossible to go fast. There were rice paddies along the road. So you couldn't really get off the road and drive because it would be muddy. And also the Vietnamese people that live there would have their gardens. And that's where their homes were—right next to the road.

Usually with a convoy of ten vehicles or so we'd have two wreckers. We'd keep those at the back of the convoy so that if somebody broke down that we would be able to repair it hopefully. I used to be a pretty good mechanic on the trucks so I could get in there and help. And then I had a couple of mechanics riding in the other truck. Each truck would have somebody that was riding shotgun—somebody with a rifle or hand grenades, a LAW[11] or something so that if we were attacked we'd be able to defend ourselves.

Well, this one particular time we were driving down the road—flat road, couldn't get off the highway because we'd get these darn trucks stuck in the mud—the Viet Cong or the North Vietnamese took us under attack. And they were using like a howitzer aiming in on our trucks. They were on the side of the road back off a couple hundred yards. They were lobbing mortar shells over in an arc and then they could see when they hit a point it would blow up. Then they'd know it would have to go five degrees this way, ten degrees that way. So they could zero in on us. In this case, they'd zero in on the convoy.

Well, I figured there wasn't much for us to do. We couldn't back up. And then, couldn't go forward. So there we were sitting there, kind of becoming a sitting duck. You know, we'd inch our way, try to the group of drivers get them off the road, get them driving up the road or someplace so that we're not just a sitting duck up there—which we were. So I would have cover of some kind. I would call in when we came under attack like that. I'd call in and request, usually what it was, was air cover. The jets would come in from Da Nang with their rockets and their machine guns. Not machine guns. Well like machine guns on the jet. Can't think of the name of it right now, but anyway I figured they'd come in from Da Nang which was behind us. We were in a little, kind of a valley. They were on the side of this hill. And they were beginning to start getting close to aiming in and getting this thing, sights set for what it would take to get us.

So I called. The Air Force runs the response. And they have spotter planes. Little two engine planes that are very maneuverable and they could get down to, you know, very tight circle. They could take a look

---

11    Department of the Army, "M-72 Series LAW, Operation and Function," Chap. 2 in *FM 3-23-25 (FM 23-25) Light Anti-Armor Weapons Field Manual*, Washington, DC: Department of the Army, August 30, 2001 and Military Factory, "M72 LAW (Light Anti-armor Weapon) Disposable Anti-tank Rocket Launcher (1963)," MilitaryFactory.com

and see what's going on. Today we do it with these remote little planes.[12] Back then we didn't have that. So this guy came in, the pilot came in and he said "Where are ya?"

Every time you go out on a convoy in an area like that you get special coordinates. So you don't actually tell the enemy where you are. But anyway, I came on the radio and I was fumbling around trying to figure out what these coordinates were. He said to me on the radio "God dammit. Just tell me where you are down there! They know where you are. They're lobbin' shells at ya. They're going to find out exactly where you are in a short time."

So he said, "Just hunker down" or something like that. And I didn't know what the hell he was talking about. I figured they were going to come in from behind us, the jets. Well, I assumed that was what they were going to do.

All of a sudden, I hear these jets coming. And they're—it looks like they're like fifty feet off the ground. But they're really they're probably a couple hundred feet off the ground. And instead of using machine gun fire or cannon fire, this guy unloads with napalm. Napalm is this tarry material that if it gets on your body it burns. It's very deadly. And the other thing is, when this stuff is shot, when it comes out, it's like syrup. And I thought *my God!* You know, if this guy is down too far down—the jet, he lobs in he's going drop it in on us. That wouldn't be good.

So fortunately they only took a few rounds to stop the Viet Cong. They got real quiet real fast. Napalm has a way of doing that. But I was—for a few minutes I was nervous—I don't like having napalm dropped in on top, above me. I think every one of us when we realized what was happening tried to dig a furrow to get out of line of sight of that napalm. Anyway, nobody got hit and eventually we continued on

---

accessed December 20, 2013, http://www.militaryfactory.com/smallarms/detail.asp?smallarms_id=72. The M-72 light anti-tank weapon or "LAW" is a shoulder-fired, disposable weapon with a collapsible tube that launched 66 mm rockets. It was used extensively in Vietnam and remains in use by the United States military in Afghanistan and Iraq.

12   Drones.

our way. That was enough excitement for one day—or two or three days actually.

## Homecoming

Coming home from Vietnam was a bit of an eye-opener. I had been in the army in Vietnam for a year at that point. And I had been at jump master school, parachute school, weapons schools. I didn't have much time off to wander around in the civilian world, but when I got back and got into the civilian world it was amazing to me the changes that had been made or went on just in the short year and a half that I was away from civilian life.

As an example, the mini-skirt. When I went into the army, if I'd have a class reunion the girls in the class would have been wearing dresses down to their ankles. When I got out of the military, came back into civilian life, women were wearing dresses just down to their butt.

And the attitude changed. I got out in Sacramento and went down to Berkeley, California where my brother was living. And this was the time of the people's party, and a lot of activism. And when I went into the army, back in the days when I hitchhiked across the United States, things like that. If you were hitchhiking it was pretty much a foregone conclusion eventually somebody was going to pick you up. But when I got back, that wasn't so. If you were wearing a uniform, I guarantee you nobody was going to pick you up.

And, you know, when I went into the army, if I went into a coffee shop when Vietnam was at the height, if I went into a coffee shop or something it wasn't unusual to offer somebody, for a complete stranger to buy me a cup of coffee and say "way to go." But then I sat back and thought about one time and realized, close to 55,000 men—especially, mainly men—were killed in the Vietnam War. And for what?

I have a daughter that was going through school and she said they had a session about Vietnam in school. In a class she was taking at Clark, Central or whatever. And I said "Oh. Well, you want some information on Vietnam? I can get you information, you know, some pictures."

And she said "Well, Daddy, we already did that. We did Vietnam this morning."

And I just thought to myself, boy. You know Vietnam warranted more than just a three hour class in the morning of a junior high school. You know, what went on? Why were we there? And, you know, 55,000 men, that's not anything to sneeze at. Wasn't anywhere near the casualties of WWI, WWII where there were hundreds of thousands, but still.

Most people don't even know where Vietnam is. Most people don't even have an inkling of why we were there.

They've never heard of Dien Bien Phu. Some of these. Dong Hoi. Khe Sanh. Da Nang. Some of these places that became hot beds of action for short periods of time. But then they just disappeared from the screen.

# DREAMS COME TRUE

# MOTORCYCLES RACING & RIDING

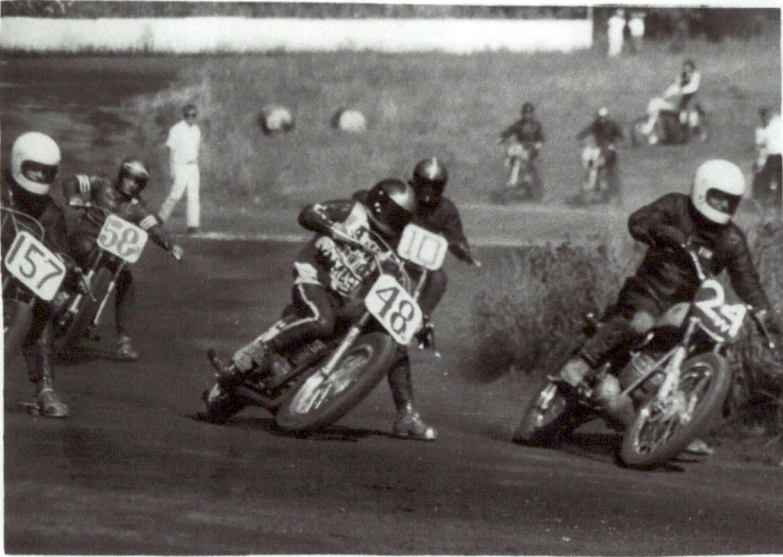

*Photo by Nancy A. Williams*

*Tim in the Lead at Sidewinders*

## Tourist Trophy

After I got out of the army I moved to Portland, Oregon and fulfilled one of my dreams - was to be involved in motorcycling - like racing. So Portland was a good area to race in because there were a lot of races going on. Like Lucky Spokes, St. Helens, Olympia, just numerous tracks all what they called "TT" — "tourist trophy." They usually had one left hand turn and a jump in it. But then that got so these race tracks didn't have a jump in any more, but they just would have a left turn. But it made for some exciting racing. Most of the tracks were surrounded by a board fence. When you missed the course and hit the board fence, it would take the wind out of your sails for a little while—to say nothing of banging your body pretty bad.

There was also something called motocross that was just coming into popularity. And that's where you go over a lot of jumps adjust tight turns. The course kind of snaked its way through areas, terrain areas — hills, gullies, trees — you name it.

Racing motorcycles was probably one of the highlights of my life. It was a lot of fun—a lot of camaraderie. St. Helens, Lucky Spokes, Sidewinders—*these were some of the tracks I raced*. There was a lot of racing going on in that part of the state of Washington, because it was just popular. A lot of young kids—sixteen, seventeen years old—could get into it and in those days you could go out and buy a motorcycle that would be competitive for around a thousand bucks. But what began to happen was motorcycles were becoming more sophisticated. When I started racing motorcycles, our front forks — at best — would have 3–4 inches of travel. So if you went over any kind of jump to speak of, a lot of times you'd get launched right off the motorcycle because there wouldn't be enough shock absorbing ability of the front forks to absorb the shock. The other thing that happened is motorcycles started getting expensive. People were using gas shocks, more sophisticated front and rear shocks, and motorcycles that would go fast.

There were enough tracks back in the late sixties that on any weekend you could go out and find a race. I probably raced about thirty times a year. The other time I'd be recuperating from a launch off the bike. But then motorcycle racing started to lose its popularity, not that it ever really had a great amount. But some of these tracks there'd be four-five hundred spectators. They would pay a nominal amount of the race. They may pay back maybe fifty percent of the earnings, of the gate. So you could make a few bucks. But it certainly wasn't enough to make a living off of.

So as the popularity of the racing community began to dwindle, I actually moved out of Portland and moved to Kennewick, Washington to start a business. And my racing days were just about over then because I lived in Kennewick and the racing was down in Portland, a hundred and eighty maybe two hundred miles away. So that became a time constraint and not being able to get to the races when I wanted to. And I had gotten to the point where if I wanted to be competitive I'd have to upgrade my equipment. That means more money into the racing program.

## Alcan

When I was getting ready to get discharged from the army after I got back from Vietnam, I was living in California. I decided to buy a motorcycle and drive it up to Alaska. I had had other motorcycles before I got into the military, but they weren't the kind of a motorcycle you could go traveling anywhere on. Matter of fact they were a motorcycle really best suited for playing in the woods and in the mud and the crud, jumping and generally ruining the bike. But anyway.

So I bought this Yamaha YZ something or other. It was a 250 cc engine in it—two hundred fifty cubic centimeters. And the bike weighed probably 300 pounds. They called it a big bear scrambler. But you had such small fork travel that you went over any kind of a jump, the bike was too stiff and it would launch you right off it. But anyway I decided it was suited for this adventure to take this motorcycle and ride to Alaska. It was combining a couple of things. I wanted to go on a trip someplace and I wanted to go to Alaska and find out about homesteading. And hoping to find entry land[13] and this was a way I would get up there and explore it.

So anyway, I got ready to leave Spokane. Loaded up my bike. I had my tent, my sleeping bag, a little bit of clothes, but I didn't have much room to carry all this and I was concerned about the weight. Turns out that when I got off the Alcan, I was coming back home, I went to a weight station in Canada on the highway and asked them if they'd weigh my bike. And they said "Sure…" So I drove on their scale and we came to the conclusion that this bike was way too heavy. It was 750 pounds for all my gear and the bike. The 250 engine was just, it was inadequate. It was okay and it was fun to drive, except that it had a top speed of about 45 miles an hour. And that would be having either a good tailwind behind you or a good hill to go down. But it was relatively dependable. I only had to rebuild the engine once on the trip. I drove it—boy I can't remember—it was a couple thousand miles anyway.

---

13    Bureau of Land Management, "BLM: Alaska: Homesteading Frequently Asked Questions," Bureau of Land Management, Department of the Interior, accessed December 11, 2013, http://www.blm.gov/ak/st/en/ prog/cultural/ak_history/homesteading/homesteading _Q_and_A.print. html. Homesteading allowed people to obtain federal land

But I went to Alaska, got as far north as Fairbanks, got down on the Kenai Peninsula. And rode on every road I could find that was rideable, and had many adventures on and off the road; to make it well worth doing. I think that the Alcan Highway is one of the best places to go on a motorcycle trip. Today the Alcan Highway is pretty well graded and paved and what not to make it a good rideable road. Pretty scenery. And you can always get gas. You have to kind of pay attention when you start. I started my trip in September. I've ridden up and down the Alcan about five, four or five times since that initial trip.

Well most of the time when I was on the Alcan with my motorcycle I was by myself. But one year this friend of mine asked me—well her son really, who was about ten, eleven years old wanted to go on a long motorcycle trip for some reason. So I said well I'm going to go down the Alcan, I'll take him with me. That should be a good adventure for him. So she said "Yeah."

When I went down the Alcan this time with Eric on the bike I had a BMW 800 cc. If I'd used that Yamaha I wouldn't have gotten anywhere. Not with him and me and all our gear on the bike. So we headed down the Alcan and for the most part the weather was good until we got to the Cassiar Highway. And it became typical Cassiar Highway weather and mud. It was pretty slimy. Had to really pay attention because you'd start slide off the road when it got really muddy. It wore me out fighting the weight, the sliding, and trying to keep the bike upright. But anyway it still was a good trip. And Eric was always finding ways to entertain himself. We had headphones, but the problem is we didn't have tape, we relied on radio. And there just aren't many radio stations along the Alcan. So he would try to read his comic books. But he'd put the comic book on my back, and then the wind would start rattling them around and ripping them apart. So that wasn't a good idea. So then I realized as we were driving down the Alcan and somebody would pass us or we'd pass somebody and the people would stare and, I thought, act kind of weird and point at him. And I didn't know what on earth was going

---

virtually free if they met requirements like living on the land and cultivating some of it. You could homestead in Alaska until October 21, 1976 when the Federal Land Policy and Management passed repealing homesteading across the United States.

on. I mean everything felt good when I turned around to look back. I couldn't see him very well because I couldn't get my head turned.

So anyway I could tell something was going on with Eric back there. Must be something going on. We had a duffle bag tied across the back of the rack on the bike, so that Eric could actually kind of sleep, hopefully. So he'd either be leaning forward with his head on my back asleep, or what I discovered what he was doing was when we went by anywhere where the sun was shining on us and creating a shadow and I looked over at the shadow beside us and saw that he was laying back on the pack, on the duffle bag, and moving his arms like a bird flying. He had his feet hooked under my legs so he was actually in there, kind of wedged in there, pretty securely. But if you just saw him, he'd look like he was going to fall off the bike.

That still worked out pretty good. In this particular trip we were going to Seattle. Finally we got down to getting close to getting off the Alcan below Fort St. John and we got into a rainstorm. And it rained. I could barely see the road so we had to pull off and wait till this rainstorm got a little bit less intense. So anyway, back on the bike we go. Finally we get down to Seattle. I asked Eric if he had fun and he wouldn't do it again. So I figured, he could still have had fun, but I don't blame him. And I did decide I'm not going to go down the Alcan again with somebody on the back of the bike, it's not much fun for them.

I only did one other bike ride where somebody was with me. And that was somebody went with me and we went around the state, circumnavigated the state of Washington. But we had the BMW and it was enough power to make it a pretty pleasant trip. And that's another good trip, is going around the perimeter of state of Washington — or at least the perimeter as much as you can get road to.

I've done a few other bike rides, but those are the only two where I've gone extensively a long ways and had somebody on the bike. The trip around the State of Washington was like a five hundred or six hundred mile trip. One thing I learned about doing some of these trips I did, especially when I was by myself. When I would pull into a campground, especially on my first motorcycle trip up to Alaska, I was somewhat of a novelty, because there weren't that many motorcycles on the highway at that time. But today there's all kinds of Yamahas, Hondas, big bikes; with radios—some of them even have televisions for the passengers, CB radios, probably internet down a lot of the highway nowadays.

What confirmed in my mind about doing what I was doing—traveling around on a motorcycle in an adventure. And this was driven home to me one time when I stopped at a campground. This couple—elderly folks, were in the campground and they had seen me before at previous places we stopped, camped out, whatever. They'd bring me extra potatoes and extra food — which was nice and I really appreciated. Anyway one night the guy, the husband, asked me about my trip and how I went about it and why and what not. I told him that I have enough money so that if this gets really erratically bad I can just take the motorcycle and sell it someplace, and buy a plane ticket, go back home. So I had a way out if I needed it. But I didn't actually think I'd ever need it.

But the point is—I realized this poor guy had worked all of his life at the post office somewhere in Nebraska. He said he realized he was always going to do this—this traveling thing. He got as far as having a real nice camper trailer and camper so he could travel in some degree of luxury. Except that he couldn't take off and hike, you know, ten miles down the road, the trail. He said he just put it off too long and then he wasn't able to do it. And I decided I didn't want to be in that position. I wanted to do it while I was still physically able to do it.

And of course as we know, or I've mentioned in these recordings elsewhere, that I've ended up with Parkinson's and that has eliminated my ability to do damn near anything. So I'm sure glad I didn't put off doing a trip on my motorcycle up the Alcan or doing an adventure like that. Because then I'd never would have been able to do it. I would have had the money to do it; but I wouldn't have the body, wouldn't have been able to physically do anything like that. Today hiking a mile or two miles is a tremendous effort. And driving a motorcycle is an impossibility. So anyway, that's what I have to live with now. But the trips that I did, especially that Alcan trip, the first one—it was just a lot of fun. The weather would get bad and I just figured I could get a hotel room if I needed to, but I don't ever remember getting a hotel room in that case. I had a wet tent a few times. But this traveling and doing these things ended up okay.

## Eagle

When I came to Alaska on my motorcycle in 19—whenever it was—'68-69, I drove of course the length of the Alcan. When I got to Tok the guy I was riding with, that I had met, wanted to go to Valdez. He had some friends who were school teachers down there. And I thought that would be cool, but first I want to go to Fairbanks and McKinley Park and as far as any other road would go. One reason I wanted to do that was when I was up in McKinley Park one day, it snowed. And it snowed about almost a foot. And I thought I want to get in all my riding and traveling around Fairbanks and this northern area, because my motorcycle and I don't deal well in snow roads.

So anyway, there was not too much exciting going on except I went into the city of Valdez. Well, what I did is, after riding all around Fairbanks, in Central and Service, the cities just outside of Fairbanks. I went across the Denali Highway. A lot of this was really scenic area and kind of a neat place to ride.

So anyway I went down to Valdez and they were just getting ready to get cranking up on the oil line. And Valdez at that time, it wasn't the madhouse that I experienced a year or two later when it was full bore construction, build that pipeline, get it done at any cost. Then the whole atmosphere of Valdez changed. It was this sleepy little village that had actually been devastated by the earthquake in '64. It had been taken over by the crowd, the people and the drinking and raising hell. There was nothing around Valdez except Valdez. So the two or three bars that were there made a hell of a killing. However, that was not exactly what I had planned on doing and wasn't too interested in hanging out with the rowdies.

So I went and got on my motorcycle and headed out. I got up to Tok which is out of Valdez 50-60 miles. And I decided I think I'll go to Eagle, because I had been told how it was really a quaint little village and it was a neat place to go. And I thought well, I can scrounge up a few days as long as it doesn't snow. So about September 10th or somewhere in there, I headed to Eagle and fell in love with the little town. There were two towns—one was the native town and one the white folks lived in. They seemed to all get along.

But there were log cabins and structures that had been built back at the turn of the century, when they were putting in the telegraph line that went from Eagle to I think eventually Valdez. This was quite a feat. One of the people in charge was a guy named Billy Mitchell, who later became famous—known for the court-martial of Billy Mitchell. He flew an airplane off of an aircraft landing ship, I don't remember what the whole story was anymore, but he was told not to do it. It was kind of ironic because now they launch stuff off the deck of these ships at random—nothing. When Billy Mitchell did this thing—it was something—enough to get him court-martialed.[14] Anyway, the people, the state government for the northern Yukon Territories had decided to rebuild some of these old structures and kind of develop more a tourist facility rather than just let these old buildings fall apart.

Dawson City was *another* town where there were a lot of miners. So the way they bought and sold things was with gold. And it became known that a good place to look for gold in these towns was in the floors of bars and whorehouses and things like that. So people were buying up these buildings and virtually gutting them out which was going to deteriorate these buildings in short order. There'd be nothing left. Now I've been up there since when they started rebuilding and it's amazing what they've done to reconstruct the area, Dawson City. And now it's kind of a tourist trap. There's a gambling casino and a honky-tonk bar and a few other things.

---

14    C. V. Glines, "William 'Billy' Mitchell: An Air Power Visionary," *Aviation History Magazine*, September 1997, republished on Historynet. com, June 12, 2006, http://www.historynet.com/william-billy-mitchell-an-air-power-visionary.htm. Gen. William "Billy" Mitchell is known as the father of the U.S. Air Force. His outspoken support of building air power versus building ships prior to WWII led in part to his court-martial. He was demoted to Colonel and remained at that rank until his death. In 1942, in the midst of WWII and six years after his death, President Franklin Roosevelt promoted him to the rank of major general (two stars) and petitioned that he be posthumously awarded the Congressional Gold Medal in recognition of his contributions to air power. The medal was awarded in 1946. While Gen. Mitchell may not have actually flown off a ship, he proposed that that is what should be done.

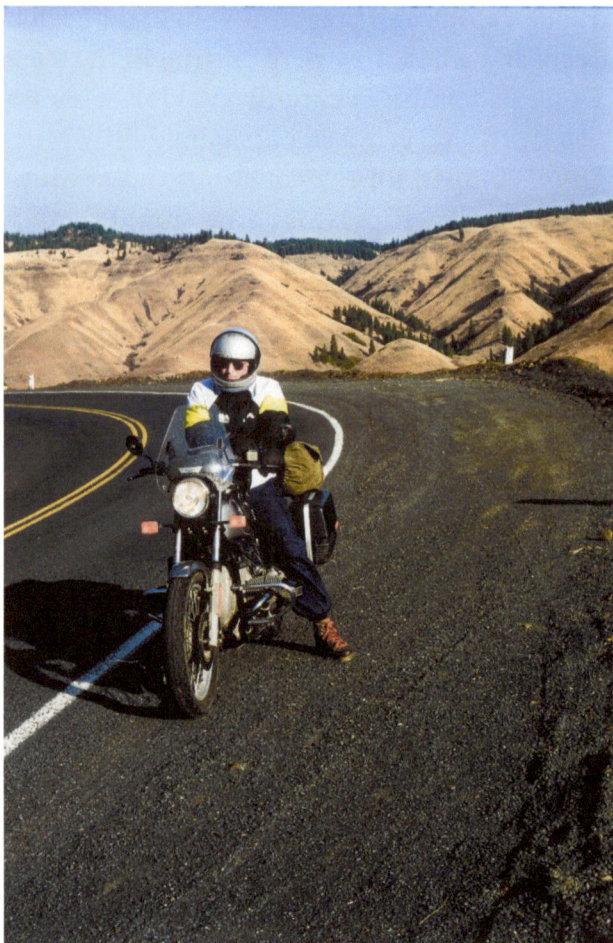

*Washington Motorcycle Trip*

## Perimeter

One great little trip I did with a friend of mine was a motorcycle trip around the perimeter of the state of Washington, camping out along the way. It's a great trip. I highly recommend it for a motorcycle. Yeah, you could do it on a bicycle too.

The trip had all the ingredients that make for a good trip. Number one I don't remember it raining. Number two the bike didn't break down. Number three it wasn't a hundred and five degrees. And number four it's pretty scenic. The other thing is that's nice for bicycle actually or motorcycle is the shoulder is wide in most places. And traffic isn't a hassle we didn't go on a weekend with something going on like speedboat races in Chelan. If they still do those. But anyway it was enjoyable. We went—I can't remember all the towns—Twisp, Methow Valley, and then we went down through Spokane. And for us it was fine because it was an opportunity to visit some friends. Then I think we went down to Lewiston, Idaho. And when we came back we went through Yakima. And that got interesting because in the Yakima Valley, especially in the orchards there are a lot of deer—whitetail deer. By the time we got someplace and got off the highway it was getting dark. And the deer started coming out. So then it became very nervous about bouncing off a deer. Which seemed to me just about happened once or twice. So anyway then we ended up over Whiteout—can't even think of the name of the pass[15], and then back to Seattle then back home.

---

15    White Pass near Naches, WA.

## SKIING

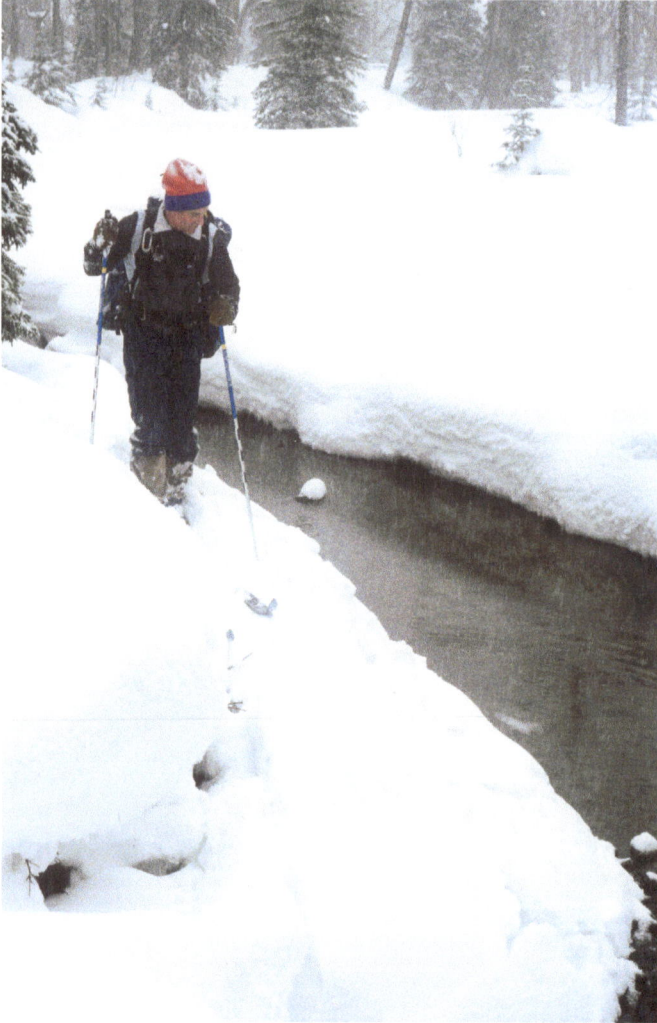

*Photo by Bonnie L. Campbell*

*Breaking Trail through Arctic Valley*

## Mt. Hood

Mt. Hood. I would have to say that Mt. Hood, which of course I forgot the elevation. It's around eleven thousand feet though I think. It's one of the best playgrounds in the mountainous area of Portland, Oregon. For one thing it's accessible. You can drive to just about every side of the mountain. There are trails up and over and down the side. There's what—three developed downhill ski areas which are all pretty, pretty fun. Well, actually Bend is in there. Bend is a different mountain, but it's close by.

I learned to ski on Mt. Hood because in the old days back about 1969–70. At two of the developed ski areas they had night skiing—under the lights. Back then it was about five bucks to ski and we'd go up there when it opened at five for night skiing. We tried to get as many runs in as we could, like maybe twenty. It wasn't a mile long run, but it was a good run.

Now Mt. Hood itself there's a ski area on the slopes and they call it the magic mile. There are two chairs. You take one chair as far as you can go, then you get off and you take another chair up. So your downhill run is about a mile. And it's just a broad ski area. About the time you start skiing the vegetation is pretty well covered; so that all the trees, brush, the shrubs, and what not are covered with snow. So I'd just make these huge turns. Go up and just do a Telemark turn that lasted for two minutes almost. You didn't have to worry about running into other people or objects.

Mt. Hood is kind of an interesting mountain. It's a volcanic mountain. I don't know the last time it blew. And I hope I don't happen to be around here when it does blow again. Its neighbor a few miles up the road is Mt. St. Helens and it did happen to blow again—made a mess of everything of course, but there was enough warning where people who were not trying to be the last guy off the mountain could make it down safely without getting hit by the ashfall or something like that.

Mt. Hood in the summertime is a great place. We used to run up there a lot. And it's a great place to do long runs. You can bike around the mountain—do a circumnavigation of the mountain. I admit that I never ended up doing that. But there are people that do it. I think they do it in a long day. But it is a nice place to ride. Wide shoulders. Laws that favor bicycle riders. It's a lot of fun, and it's worth recreating on.

It can get bad weather up there. They get whiteout conditions and people have been lost. They don't know which way up is because they're up there on this broad ski slope. You can go a mile in one direction and a mile in another direction there's nothing but snow out there. So people lose their orientation as to where they are, get lost, and wander off. And it used to be every couple of years, seems like, somebody would die. They have avalanche problems also.

People have done a lot of different things that have become a first ever type thing. Some guy skied off the top of Mt. Hood on about seven- or eight-foot-long skis. It's pretty amazing. There's an old park ranger that in his career in living and working on Mt. Hood, that has been up and over the peak over 650 times. He did this so much they decided that they wanted to build a lookout on top of Mt. Hood, a fire lookout. It does have a pretty good view, a 360 degree panoramic view—there's not much blocking *the view* for a fire lookout. Anyway this guy ended up hauling up timbers and wood and stuff enough to make a fire lookout. One of the problems is, it snows so much up there that things get buried in the snow and can get damaged. Of course his lookout would just be covered by snow and nothing would happen to it. Although in later years it disappeared because of the high winds. Mt. Hood is one of these peaks like Valdez getting 300 inches of snow—amazing.

# GOING HIGH

# MOUNTAINEERING

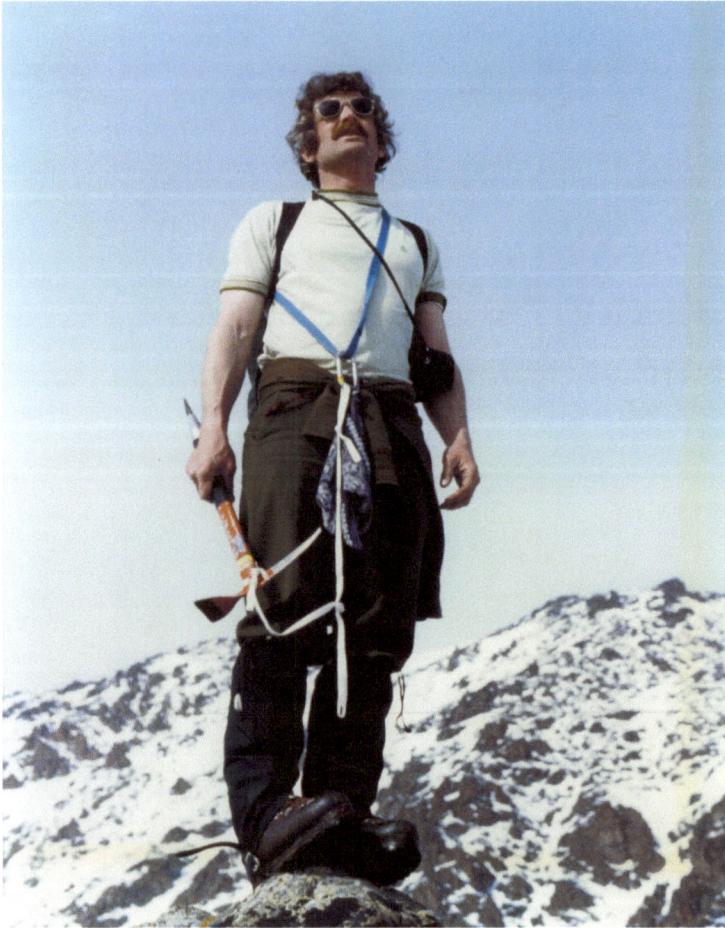

*Photo courtesy Tim Neale*

*Climbing in the Chugach*

## Mountaineering Club of Alaska

So how did I get into mountain climbing? Slowly. When I moved to Alaska in 1970 or so, I decided I wanted to get into climbing and do more hikes. When I was living in Spokane I did some of this, but in Spokane the climbing was mainly rock climbing, technical climbing. I looked into the best way do this and found a company called Mountain Trip had mountaineering classes and that type of thing. They led certain climbs and certain travel trips. I did a few of those and with Mountain Trip went into the Chugach range and did O'Malley, the Ramp, and the Wedge and all these peaks in the front range.[16] And I decided this is something I want to do. I had thought of getting into canoeing and kayaking, because I had more of a background or did more of that type of thing when I was in the Spokane than I did the mountaineering thing. To do mountaineering or glacier stuff you'd have to go across the state to Mount Rainier and that was 300 miles away. There was no ice climbing and no glacier travel because there's none around Spokane. There was some good rock climbing in the area, but it was too far from any permanent snow fields to get in to much snow or ice climbing.

So anyway I got involved in the mountaineering club and began to participate in activities. There was a fairly good sized group of people involved in mountaineering at that time, because for one thing it was a good opportunity for people that just came to Alaska to go to these mountaineering club meetings and meet other people with like interests. Eventually, I became president of the club along with a few other notable climbers of past years, but the big thing was each year the club would put on an ice climbing school up at Matanuska glacier. That was usually a three day event. It was a lot of fun. And a lot of people got involved in mountaineering, ice climbing, and scrambling.

During my career of being in the Mountaineering Club of Alaska I had a lot of great times and some not so great. But I used to do a climbing class, a basic climbing class. *One of the things we practiced was* ascending a rope. If they fell in a crevasse, they'd be able to ascend a rope to get out. Well it was a lot easier to ascend a rope that was in my back yard. We could be there sitting and drinking a beer and watching the students discover how hard it was to ascend a rope when you've got sixty, seventy pounds on your back and trying use these ascenders and make any progress.

To ascend a rope you use the infamous jumars which just clamp onto the rope. You just push one ascender up and alternate pushing one, pushing the other. Push them up and lift your foot. You've got to lift your foot, lift your leg, so that there's slack in the rope to ascend. And definitely you can see how difficult it becomes. People that climb

---

16    The "front range" of the Chugach Mountains outside of Anchorage, Alaska.

a lot know what it's like to fall in a crevasse. It's not fun. Can be scary. Plus you have a bell shaped crevasse that doesn't allow you to reach the side of the crevasse to help you get up. You put your foot and try to ascend up, and it's just difficult. I discovered it was much easier to do this on one of the trees in my front yard, than it was to go up to the Matanuska glacier or go up to a real glacier someplace and try to ascend. Ascending a rope doesn't come natural. It can be a difficult task at best depending upon how much weight you've got.

I've only fallen in a couple *crevasses* where it was exciting. Most of my experiences were to find the crevasse with a probe or an ice axe before crossing the area where there probably was a crevasse under the snow. So the big clue I always had was stay out of them. They can be very dangerous. There have been several people killed not paying attention to check for crevasses. Some people go along and never fall in a crevasse in their life. Yet they've walked on ice fields for miles. But if you're foolish enough, I shouldn't say foolish, if you're out on a glacier traveling around an you're the only one out there and you fall in a crevasse, well that can be disconcerting. So no matter where you are in your learning about mountaineering, you need to practice these skills and use them. You don't want to be out there in a crevasse field and go through a crevasse that's perpendicular to where you're traveling. You end up tipping over with your head down and your butt up. If you're traveling across a glacier generally you've got a pack on. Hopefully you can somehow wiggle out of that pack. Let it fall down, *but still be* attached to your pack. Get rid of that weight off your back somehow.

*In a* class, where you go hang off a tree, you *can* learn these things in a big hurry. *Beginners have* got to have an idea of how difficult or hard it is to do some of these maneuvers. Right off the top of my head, which is not all that good these days, but I'd say that falling into a crevasse is one of the more major accidents that you can find yourself in and not be able to do something about it. *For* climbing, four is a good number. One is not a good number. Also it's better to do your training and practicing, and learning how to use your jumars, your ascenders, your rope *in a class. That way* you know how you get roped up to the person ahead of you so you can get out of the rope if need be — all these skills. There's a book out — I can't think of the name of it right now. But it's a Seattle mountaineering book that they published years ago and update periodically.[17] And it gives you all kinds of ideas about how to handle crevasses, how to handle a lot of things. I've got to go get the book.

## First Big Climb

My first big climb was Mt. McKinley[18] with Mountain Trip[19]. And that was a real experience because although it was a guided trip, everybody pitched in—like buying and packing the food, making sure everybody had the right number of ascenders and crampons and some kind of warm boots—although most of us used the infamous white bunny boots. But they're not exactly friendly after you've been climbing for a couple weeks and they're hanging out with your dirty old feet in them. But anyway, that's another story.

So our climb was to go up one side and come down the other side. Go up the Kahiltna and come out at Wonder Lake. And that was a good trip. It was enjoyable. Didn't have any major problems. But when we did get off the mountain, I had a friend that was going to run the Mayor's Marathon the next day. And I had encouraged her to start running and quit smoking and get physically fit and so she did. And it worked out as almost overlapping my climb on McKinley. She ended up running the Marathon the day after I got back. So I had a desire to get back and catch her to cheer her on as she was running the race in Anchorage, the Mayor's Marathon. But I didn't quite get back in time. So I got out to Wonder Lake and I pushed ahead of the rest of the group of people in my group that had climbed the mountain. So I essentially got up there a few hours before anybody else did. Anyway, the park ranger came

---

17   Harvey Manning, ed., *Mountaineering: Freedom of the Hills*, Seattle: The Mountaineers, 1960.

18   E. J. R. David, "Why it's time to (finally) officially rename Mount McKinley as Denali," *Alaska Dispatch*, February 12, 2013. Mount McKinley is often referred to as Denali, an Athabascan word meaning "The Great One." Efforts to rename it continue to this day.

19   Mountain Trip telephone conversation Jan 28, 2014. Although it is now owned by others, the mountain guiding service Mountain Trip was established in Alaska in 1973 by Tim's friend Gary Bocarde.

over and saw me because I looked like a climber—the grunge look. Probably didn't smell too sweet.

We were going to go and take the train back to Anchorage. So the first thing the guy told us was to go ahead and order a meal on the train. So we ordered a meal and scarfed that down. Then he said "Well, if you want to have another meal. We'll pay for it." And of course, after eating freeze dried food, and then we ran out of food on the climb. And kind of starving ourselves, it was like having a home cooked meal on the train. So we availed ourselves of the opportunity to eat something that wasn't freeze dried, and that tasted good, and was fresh.

So that's basically how I got started with climbing. Then I went on to climb some other peaks like Mt. Hood, Mt. Drum, Mt. Sanford, Pioneer peak, and mountains like that in the front range of the state park here.

## McKinley

*Memory is a fragile thing. Tim's first big climb came in the late 1970s/early 1980s. Parkinson's makes dates, names, and places once at the tip of the tongue elusive. To aid Tim in recollecting his first big climb, his home aid Jesus Torres asked him questions while they reviewed a slide show Tim had shown of his adventure.*

So here we are getting prepared to go climb Mt. McKinley. I believe that was the summer of 1983. Again accuracy of these dates and things is a little suspect, but anyway we'll try to do the best we can. This was a group of people that signed up with Gary Bocarde to do this trip. At that time his business was Mountain Trip. A good claim to fame he has for his initial business guiding up the mountain was to take four hang gliders up McKinley and then they were going to fly off the top of McKinley and down to the Kahiltna glacier or wherever they thought as far as they could get. But that didn't have anything to do with our climb. That was the year before, a year or two before our climb.

We used a van to haul the food up there. We actually started out from Talkeetna and flew into the Kahiltna glacier. So we didn't have to carry all the food from this point on our backs.

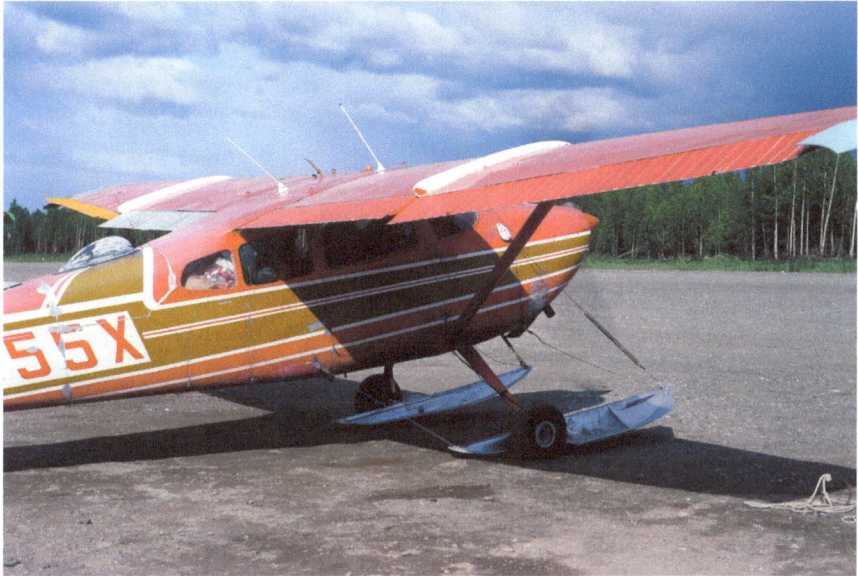

*Flight to Kahiltna*

In those days the safety rules were somewhat suspect because the object here was to get as much gear on the mountain with each flight. And that's exactly what this was. Just stuff it all in there so that the plane will get off the ground and take it into Kahiltna glacier where our base camp was.

Notice the wheel skis. They use the wheel skis on the ground, dirt. Then as soon as they get up in the air they pump the hydraulics to lower the skis so that when you land on the glacier you're on snow.

Well we're heading towards the mountain. We're going into the Kahiltna glacier. McKinley's up there someplace. Gets to be a little more snow the further we go there. One-shot pass. You come flying in there and it looks like you're going to come in and hit the pass. You're too low. You get up close to there and the air is coming from back on the mountain there and what it does it gives you uplift, whatever they call that. Anyway the plane just lifts up, shoots over the pass and there you are. When you're flying in it seems like you're closer to the mountains than you want to be. But on the other hand you hope these pilots know what they're doing, and they've been around long enough that they obviously, probably do.

### Kahiltna — first camp at 7400'

Well, we parked the plane on that glacier, because most of the people that climb McKinley climb it starting from the Kahiltna. We were starting on the Kahiltna, but we were going over to the Muldrow which is on the other side of the mountain. Come out at Wonder Lake.

The Kahiltna, unloading all that stuff and establishing a base camp. It's 6,500' so we've got to climb up to 20,000' on McKinley. Drag all that stuff with us. Base camp, actually *there's* a radio antenna there. In the days before cell phones and what not, different guides and the different air taxi services would put up a tent and this lady would kind of be an air traffic control person at the base camp. But it was a way of communicating, letting people know if a plane is coming in or having some kind of a problem. And she kind of keeps track of the groups and where they are.

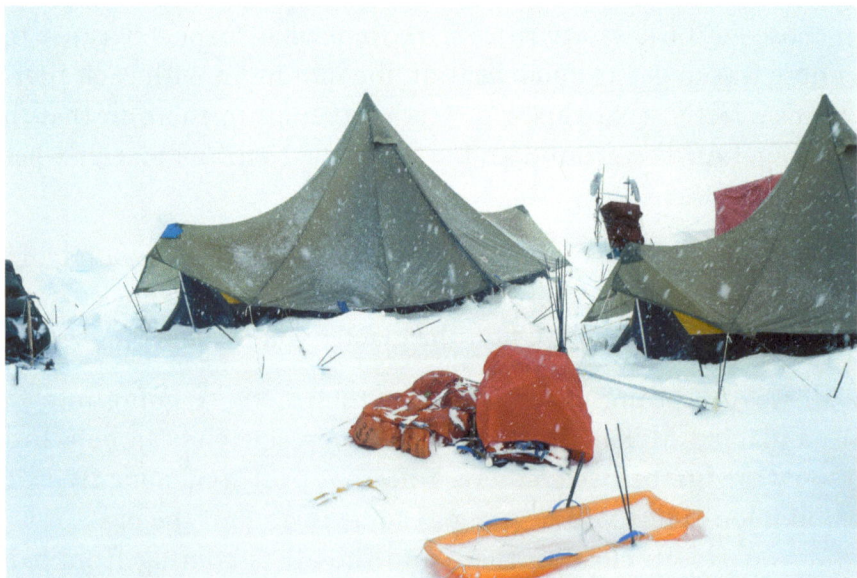

*Tents on McKinley (with bamboo poles, frame packs, and wands)*

Photo courtesy Tim Neale

There can be darn near 30 people here in this base camp. There were 10 of us in the group I was with. There was Jim Hale, can't think of the guy's name now. Actually there were only a couple of us from

Alaska and the rest were from California. Most of them knew each other. That was kind of the reason there was such a big group on one climb. Anyway there are two or three guided groups that are in this same area. Starting out it gets kind of busy out there. We put everybody in two tents — *big, old pointy tents*. I use dome tents now. Matter of fact the only time I used these tents was on this climb.

Most everybody on this trip used these white, we call them in Alaska "bunny boots." But they were actually designed and used in Korea. And they're really like a rubber boot, they're insulated. So you don't need to worry about freezing your feet in them, unless it's really cold. The problem is you can get foot rot in them because they don't breathe. Every time I got to where we camped, after we set up camp, I'd take my bunny boots off and walk around in the snow a little bit; to kind of wash the boots and wash my feet so they didn't smell so bad.

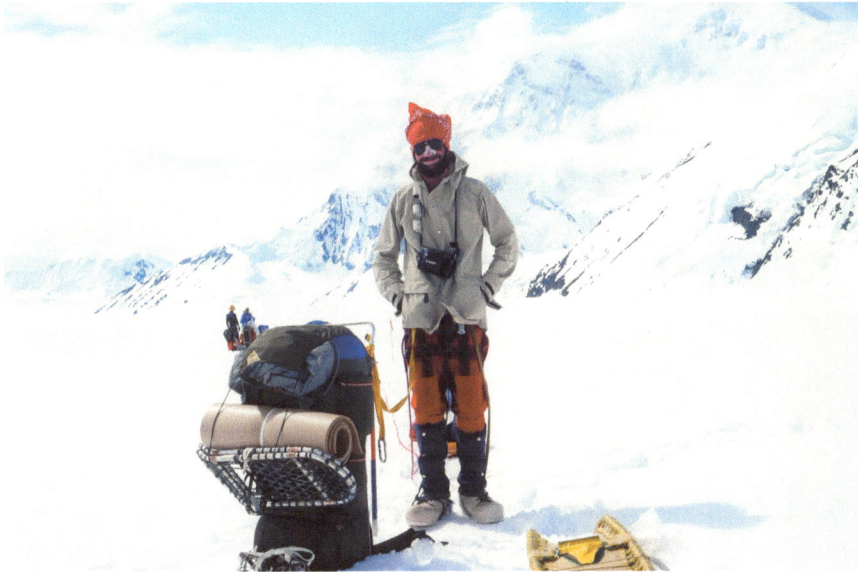

*Photo courtesy Tim Neale*

*Tim Ready to Climb Mt McKinley*

No this actually isn't a woodchuck this is me. And I think we've got our bunny boots on and our super dark sunglasses. Back then they seemed to have two grades of sunglasses. You'd either have something you could see out of or these sunglasses that I've got. They're so dark you can't really see what's going on. On the other hand it's better than having sunburned eyes.

*Going without a shirt like I did,* now that's another thing that's very foolish. You can get scorched by that sun because there's not the UV protection *up there* — so I learned later. Well I knew when I was living on the ranch you know, your skin would just get cooked. Get out there in that sun all day long. But here it's reflecting off the snow. You put this zinc stuff that about 100% block of the sun, because you can really get scorched. Especially up at this elevation where you don't have much UV protection from the sun.

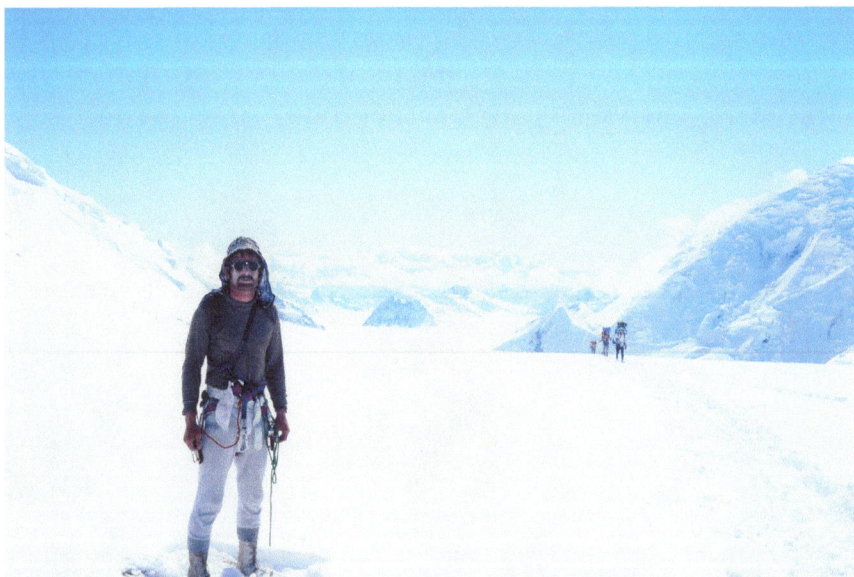

Snowshoeing on McKinley

*Photo courtesy Tim Neale*

Well I'll tell you how ancient this is. My long underwear is cotton long underwear. Now everything is polypropylene. Some of this stuff, like what I *wore*, some will use wool long underwear. One of the problems with the stuff like I *wore* is it gets wet and it doesn't dry out. Polypropylene dries out. It doesn't smell very good, but at least you can stay warmer than if you have wool long underwear, it gets damp and it gets cold. But once you start gaining altitude your clothes will dry because the air is so dry. *The moisture just gets sucked out.* Actually essentially it evaporates.

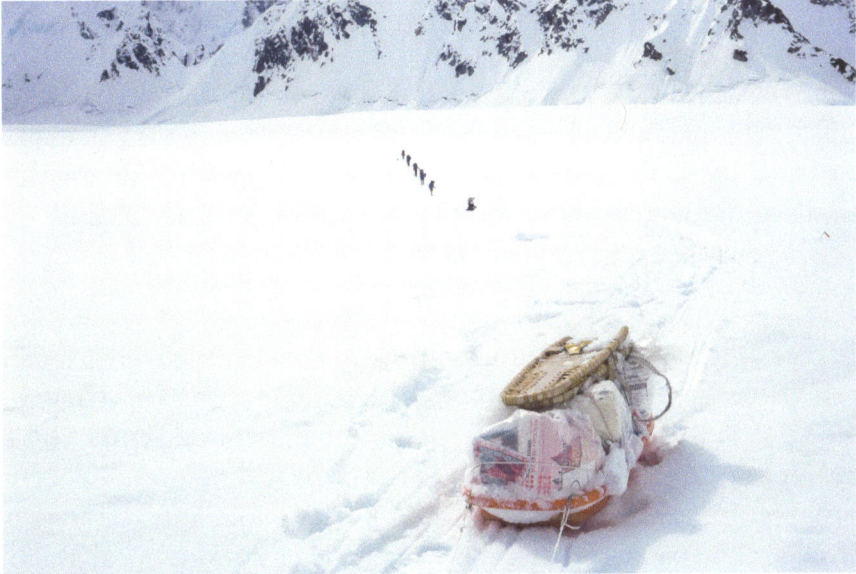

*Photo courtesy Tim Neale*

*Sleds on McKinley*

Loading stuff up, these little orange sleds are one of the best things going for hauling. Even doing a trip back in the Chugach for two or three days it's handy to use one of these little sleds. Gary and I and another guy we got up to camp at 14,000'. And we were transferring loads so we took a load up there and dropped it off, and then we had to go back down and get another load. And we decided that we'll take these sleds down with us. Each of us would have a long, a couple mile long sled ride. That was about the only time we ever did that.

So this time we used snowshoes. The trouble with using skis is everybody has to be able to ski at somewhat the same speed. And that's not always very possible. So it's easier using snowshoes. Plus if you're going along like you do on McKinley and most other mountains there are times when you need crampons. So, if you've got skis on it's kind of a hassle to take them off and put skis on. With the snowshoes, they've got little cleats on under the sole. They're designed to give a little traction on the ice. So you can get by with using those as opposed to taking the snowshoes off and putting on crampons, taking the crampons off and putting on snowshoes.

You're towing a load and then you've got the load that's on your back. And when you look at that you've got to remember that if you fall in a crevasse with all this stuff on you, it's going to be a monumental effort to get back out of there. Usually what you do is you tie on that sled onto your rope so that if you do fall into a crevasse you can jettison that load there. And have it on like parachute cord or webbing twelve- or fifteen-feet-long. It's hard to explain so I probably won't try to explain it. But basically you've got to get away from that pack or that load. But you don't want to jettison into the bottom of the crevasse, because your food that you're going to need has to be on there and *you want to* be able to recover it.

Bamboo ski poles and aluminum frame packs. We were all using ski poles because they're a good tool to probe for crevasses. They were bamboo poles, which used to be a kind of pole that everybody uses for all kinds of skiing. Ancient equipment. This is just before they started to manufacture these soft packs. *They're* more like a duffle bag, but they fit your body a little better than an aluminum frame pack. You had more places to adjust. Initially people used wood packs which didn't fit your body very much. Then these aluminum framed packs came out and they became very popular. And then soft packs like I *used*. People in California and Colorado started to develop climbing gear realized there was a market for it. So this stuff gets upgraded. For ten or fifteen years there—almost constantly—there was something new coming out on the market. New material *for example*—so you wouldn't have a lot of weight in your pack and frame and all that.

### Ned and Galen

The summit of McKinley looks like you could just take off and trot right up the mountain. While we were on the mountain climbing there were two guys Ned Gillette and Galen Rowell who were *attempting* a one day try to climb Mt. McKinley, *coming* down the Kahiltna.

*Sprinting? Running off it? No, nobody runs up there.* No, these guys—they had emergency gear. They got up to the top and by the time they were coming down we were up at 14,000 about and saw them walking down. Ned Gillette had Galen Rowell on about a five-foot rope. Galen suffered from pulmonary edema, having problems breathing, his lungs are clogged. And Ned Gillette, the next morning Ned looked like one of us. However Ned Gillette was an Olympic skier at some point a few years ago. So he's got a well-conditioned body. And Galen Rowell is a professional photographer. When he got down to us—they didn't have sleeping bags, so we just put him inside. We put him in a tent and gave him liquids and some food. But the main thing they needed was liquids. Don't know what would have happened if we hadn't been there. There weren't exactly a lot of people climbing at that point. And besides that a lot of people a lot of guided groups and people climbing on their own could possibly get a little stressed out. So they were using all the energy they had to take care of themselves. So the next morning we waved goodbye to Ned Gillette and Galen Rowell and wished them luck. And they took off heading down and we took off heading up.

Some of the crevasses are open. Sometimes I think I'd rather be going through crevasses that are open or just a blank glacier where there doesn't appear to be any crevasses, but they're still out there they can gobble you up if you're not careful. A lot of them you can't see, or if it's been blowing and the surface all looks the same. That can get kind of spooky. Avalanches come off some of that stuff *too*. They're not big avalanches, but they're avalanches. And they have the potential. So you've got to be careful, because if the crevasse doesn't get you the avalanche will.

Every time you move, in theory if I remember this correctly, which I think I do, you climb up. During one day you spend climbing up. You haul as much as you can climbing up, and then you drop your load, go back down. Just kind of keep relaying loads. Especially when you go over the top of the mountain, you have to take more gear than you would if you were going up to McKinley and then turning around and just going back down. But if you go over the top, in theory you've got to have enough food and fuel to take you down the other side. And it doesn't do any good to cache food there because you're not going to go back and get it. Although some of these guided groups, if they have hauled stuff up and cached it and decided they can't go back up and get it, they'll let somebody else use their food and fuel rather than just let it go to waste.

Oh and here's another thing—putting in wands. Later in the year, the park service goes up there I understand. I haven't seen it. But they go up there and mark a route off with wands to help. Because if it gets windy up here, which it can. *At this point, between 10,000' and 11,000',* we've been really lucky. We haven't had a storm. This is about in May. *In photos* I notice there's no wind blowing. I'm sitting without a jacket on.

## Breaktime

We make up packs for breakfast and for dinner and then for lunch we just have these bags *with* a candy bar and a bag of gorp. Actually what you do is you get your bag of gorp, make that up in the morning and everybody may be entitled to a cupful of gorp and freeze dried fruit and things like that. Then you'd just dole it out to yourself. So you see when we stop, people bent over. Usually they're digging in and grabbing their food. This is getting to be the point where you're hungry. So this goes in stages. As a matter of fact you're hungry because you get hungry once you start, *and have* been out there hiking around for two or three days. You get tired and your energy level goes up and down, but you want more food. So you want to eat more. And then you climb up and you get to the top.

Then the next thing that happens is you get to the top and lack of oxygen and you start getting sick from altitude. So then you don't want to eat anything. You don't even want to hear the word food. And that can become a problem, because if you're going up and over the top you know you have got to haul your food. So what we did up there is say "okay here's all the food we have" and laid it out on a tarp or something. And then everybody could go in there. We doled out the candy bars and juices—powder, mixed. Just let people take whatever food they wanted. And of course everybody is either half sick or all the way sick.

Then the next thing is all that rope laying there. You've got to deal with that rope. When you stop you've got to try not to get it knotted up. Don't cross the other *ropes*. There's probably three rope teams there. *If the teams don't* think about what they're doing, *the ropes can get all knotted up.*

## Joe

Joe Mirra was a brain surgeon. He and I were good buddies in the climb. We buddied up. Usually you pair up with somebody—two or three of you. Of course nowadays with my brain problems I could have my own doctor coming along next time. We made the summit and came back down and we were climbing down. We stopped for a break. Joe was lying on the snow and I went over to ask him if he was okay, and I see this red liquid coming out of his mouth. And I said "Joe! Are you okay, what's the matter?"

And he said, "Tim, you idiot. I just mixed up some red drink. That's my liquid, I'm not bleedin'!"

"Oh, okay. Good Joe. Thanks for telling me."

We all got a good laugh about that.

Joe Mirra, good guy. Brain doctor. Yeah I wish I could see him now.

### Cache at 13000'

*At 13,000', we had a cache.* This is the place where we'd go up and dump one load. Go back and pick up another and haul it up. Just kind of relay our supplies up as best we can. One thing that we discovered you have to be careful of is that the ravens were flying this high on the mountain. Which normally they don't fly this high, but they say that the ravens are able to go higher on the mountain than you'd normally would find them because they're just getting into these caches and eating their way up. So you've got to be sure if you cache, that you do something to mitigate the ability of the ravens to get in there and have lunch on your expense. Dig them deep enough or get snow or something over them.

We were relaying loads up and one of our team people there was getting too tired to make another load up to the cache from down below. So Gary had this person stay in camp and the rest of us would go up. This person was supposed to have all the stoves cooking away so we could boil enough water because we were pretty low on extra water. So we were thinking we were going to have all kinds of water when we got there. You're always dehydrated and you need to hydrate as much as possible. Some people feel that being hydrated kind of keeps the mountain sickness away. *But* this person went in and laid down in the tent apparently. *By the time* we got *back,* they'd let the stoves run out of fuel. This is when you stop and take a break then you're normally eating your lunch which is gorp, cheese, pieces of crackers. Then you mix up some Gatorade or something to give you a little bit of a bump there.

### Storm Day camp 3. Relaying loads

About 15,000' is getting up where we begin thinking we've got a ways to go. We're eventually going to get up, cache all our food that we're hauling. Because we're going to summit, come back down to this point on the mountain somewhere about 18–19,000' divide up all the food we've got left and we're going to hike out to Wonder Lake.

*Between 14,000 and 16,000' you go around Windy Corner. It's* another one of these days where it's windy, not much visibility; you're beginning to feel the effects of altitude. At 14,000' I personally begin to start feeling rotten from the altitude. *It doesn't look inviting. It's grueling.* That's why I have no desire to go up there anymore. Once was enough.

### Fixed line to 16,000'

The park service usually puts in a fixed line at this point. Because people like us we're going to ferry loads up this slope. And it's pretty *steep*—it's a couple thousand feet. So they have this fixed line in there and anchored off. You stay roped in to your team members, but you put in a jumar or some kind of an ascender on this fixed rope and use that *as protection*. Basically it's steep and if you slide you know you'd go a long ways. And that's one reason why the fixed line is good and it's pretty well anchored down there. But you still want to be anchored into your team. It's hard to tell, but it is actually pretty steep up there.

### 17,000'

This is about where we encountered Galen Rowell and Ned Gillette on their attempt to do a one day ascent of McKinley. And somewhere it had to be flat, because I slept outside the tent. I slept in a bivvy bag, because people were snoring and it was crowded in the tent. So I was laying out there *outside*. I think I was anchored in. And I hear this squeaking noise of somebody walking in snow, crunching their way up. And it's about, probably—I'm just going to guesstimate—probably somewhere about 4 o'clock in the morning. Somebody comes up to me and says "What are you doing up here?"

And I said "Well, I'm trying to get some sleep, the tent's crowded."

And they said "Who you with?"

And I told him. This guy says "Bocarde, is that you in there in the tent?"

And Bocarde says "Hey Galen, is that you?"

They recognized each other. Of course both of them were pretty good rock climbers in their own right at Yosemite. And I think I mentioned before about Galen Rowell and Ned Gillette. *Galen was a photographer.* Ned Gillette was an adventurer, he'd do long trips. He did a circumnavigation of McKinley—he went all the way around it, but at the base of it. It wasn't totally unusual that *these two guys found each other on the mountain,* because this is where these guys play. However, one sad story, I was reading the paper a while back and read that Ned Gillette and his wife were killed by bandits in Pakistan or someplace.[20] And I think, I'm not sure, but I think Galen Rowell was killed in a plane accident someplace[21]. But you can find, if you googled Galen Rowell, you'd see some great photographs that he's taken—especially in Yosemite. Being a rock climber himself, he could get up on some of these rock faces and be taking pictures. Get some pretty impressive stuff.

### 17,000' to Denali Pass

Well Denali Pass is where we do the cache the last time, because we're going to go down from here. At this point we do the summit and then go back down to Wonder Lake.

---

20    Jesse Cassidy, "The Story of 'Historical Badass' Ned Gillette | From Skiing Earth's Highest Summits to Being Shot to Death in Pakistan," *Snow Brains*, June 26, 2013, http://snowbrains.com/ned-gillette/; Michael Frank, "Historical Badass: Climber, Skier, Adventurer Ned Gillette," *Adventure Journal*, December 5, 2012, http://www.adventure-journal.com/2012/12/historical-badass-climber-skier-adventurer-ned-gillette/. Ned Gillette and his wife were shot in their tent in the Karakoram on August 4, 1998. Although his wife survived, Gillette died the next morning.

Among his many adventures, he'd circumnavigated Mount McKinley (Denali) in 1978 and a couple weeks later by made the first one-day ascent with Galen Rowell that Tim references.

21    Mountain Light, "Mountain Light Press Release Monday, August 12, 2002," Moutainlight.com, August 12, 2002, http://mountainlight.com/PR.html. Galen and his wife Barbara Cushman Rowell were killed in a plane crash near the airport in Bishop, California while returning home from a workshop on August 12, 2002. Their photographs continue to be sold through the business they began in 1983.

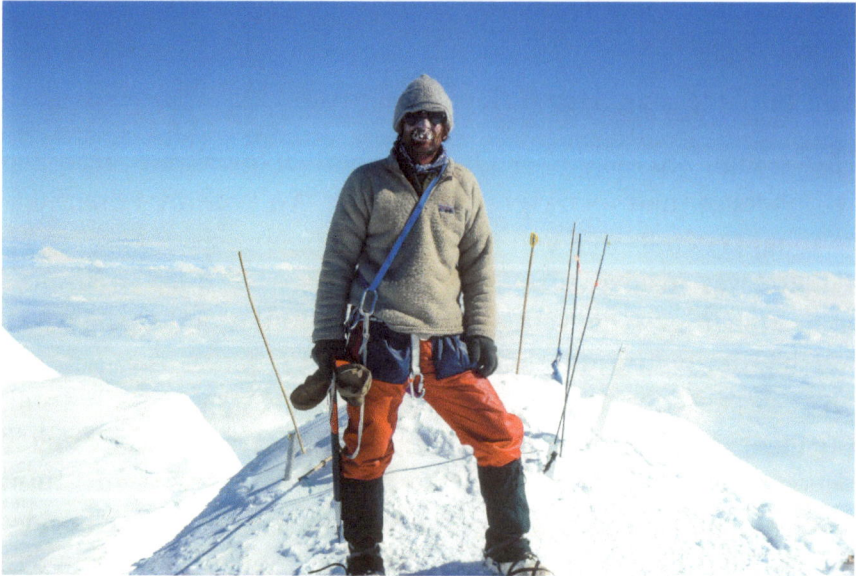

*Photo courtesy Tim Neale*

*Tim on the Summit of McKinley*

**Summit**

The summit—I took this shot so I could prove I was there. No register. The wands let you know where the summit is. One thing we got was good weather. *It was* a good summit day because you could see. And I think we got all 10 people to the summit if I recall correctly. It *was* pretty cold and windy, because I had my wind pants on and I had my fuzzy jacket. My pile jacket I only wore when it was getting considerably below freezing.

*From the summit you could see* Mount Foraker at 17,000'. Some clouds were coming in *below us. We'd climbed through them and couldn't see anything.* If it's like storm days when you can't see—if you don't have any visibility, you have no business out there climbing around because you can step off of something. I mean if you stepped off, that wouldn't be good. *Anyway, it* looked like something building up. These mountain storms they can blow up from one side of the mountain to the other. You can be in perfect weather almost twenty minutes later you're engulfed in clouds and storm.

There's a north and a south peak. North peak is a peak that people don't climb much. I can't remember the difference in elevation between the two peaks, but people want the highest peak so they're going to go for the south. *The north peak isn't particularly dangerous; it just doesn't get climbed as much.*

A point of trivia, and I think I've got this piece of trivia correct. Years and years ago these guys climbed the mountain and they climbed the north peak. They hauled up a twelve-foot birch pole—a twelve-foot-high birch log you might say, and planted it up on the north peak thinking that you can see Fairbanks. They wanted people to be able to see that they'd climbed the mountain. So they could see from Fairbanks—see this twelve-foot-high pole. Well it didn't work. *You* couldn't see it.[22]

*The pole of course is no longer there.* At this elevation stuff that's stuck up there, not stuck up there, but caches and people that discard gear and everything. It doesn't deteriorate, you know, it stays. Actually becomes petrified actually which is causing a problem. People that climb they leave their human waste up on the mountain which you'd expect. But they're getting to be so many people climbing the mountain now that their human waste is becoming a kind of a danger for contamination. So the National Park Service has had a couple of expeditions up there to haul as much of that waste off the mountain as they can. And a matter of fact, I think now you can't just dig a hole in the snow and use it for your toilet. You've got to, if you have toilet paper and poop, you've got to haul it back down with you. *A difficult task*, but something has to be done about it. It's not a big area. The total area where you can hang out or set up a camp or whatever isn't that large. So you get up there where you get a thousand people tromping through there camping and what not. I don't know how many people climb the mountain. I guess I should look that one up. But it's a lot.

My recollection of the summit was—boy it was cold up there. And this time we head back down we don't have tents set up that we were going come back down to like when we were hauling the caches up and down, and up and down. At least when it got real cold during the day when we were hauling and we come back down to our camp we

22   Barry O'Flynn, "The Sourdough Expedition to Mount McKinley" Irish Mountaineering Club, September 2007, http://www.irishmountaineeringclub. org/index.php?option=com_content&task=view&id=128&Itemid=89. Tim is referring to what is known as the "Sourdough Expedition." In 1910, four local Alaskans ("sourdoughs")

had tents all set up and can jump in them. But here we didn't have any tents set up.

### Summit Tangles

Well here's another thing that becomes a problem is this rope kind of strewn around here. You should always think — if you're climbing and there's more than one of you — you've got a rope. You've got to think of rope discipline. For one thing, you've got crampons on you don't walk on the rope or in the tent with crampons. And you'd be surprised how many people would be out there standing around, look down and *hear* "Get off the rope with your crampons!" But the other thing is tangles. It's just aggravating. Somebody might come along and walk over, cross over, these ropes are laying there and then they get them tangled. And then you've got to untangle them. That's why you keep usually three people — four in this case — to a rope. And when you stop you leave the rope stretched on the ground. Everybody doesn't come back and hang out like this. What has happened here is people have walked back and forth, and you shouldn't walk around up there without a rope on.

### Heading Off the Mountain

At this point all anybody wanted to do was get down in elevation. One thing it'd be warmer, but the other thing you could breathe easier. This is also where we set out a tent, laid it out on the snow flat, took all the food that we had left, and spread it out on the tent. Then we started dividing it up. People could go in and get a chocolate bar *or something*. It was all laid out there, but not organized very well. There might be some freeze dried oatmeal packets or something like that. And there were always soup packets, because soup is so easy to make once you get the stoves going. That's why it was such a bummer when that person left our stoves on, and let them run out *of fuel when we were carrying loads and caching them on the way up the mountain. When* we got back and we had nothing but cold water and not much of that. Had the stoves kept going until we got there, someone else could take over the stoves, and we would have had several quarts of water.

---

from the Kantishna mining district — Tom Lloyd, Billy Taylor, Pete Anderson, and Charles McGonagall — summited McKinley's lower north peak and placed a spruce flagpole noting their achievement. While many doubted their success, expedition leader Hudson Stuck verified their climb in 1913 seeing the pole en route to the south summit.

Also at this point if I recall correctly, and I think I am correct on this. We started out with seven MSR stoves or something to that effect. And ended up with when we were up here I think we had one that worked, marginally. Maybe two, but I think it was one. Any time we stopped we had to have that stove going so we could have some kind of water. Because it was going to be a while before we got off the mountain far enough to get water out of the lakes or streams or whatever we hoped had the least amount of giardia in it.

### Harpers Glacier

*On the way down you'd see* some rope hanging up. Here you'd see a piece of rope, maybe up there there's some rope, and you wonder what's that from? Well, that's from earlier climbs. Some of them go back to the original people that tried to climb this mountain. You'd think it would disappear with age, but it doesn't. It's just like petrified and its preserved there. Probably they didn't want to haul them back. You know, they were done. These early guys, you know, you wonder how they ever survived — the weather, altitude, falling in a crevasse. They are some good books on McKinley climbing. Like "Hall of the Mountain King" and "White Winds". "Hall of the Mountain King" was written by a guy named Schneider and he was involved in the worst disaster as far as deaths on the mountain ever. I think there were six or seven of them died. Pretty sad.

Coming down through Harper's glacier looks pretty uninviting, but it's relatively easy to get through the icefall. There were crevasses up around the ice blocks, but if you send somebody down there looking for a route that knows something about crevasses and knows how to read snow you can do it. Gary was on a rope coming down through there and he was leading, picking out a route. Gary and I were pretty good buds and he had me right behind him. All of a sudden, my rope went tight going to Gary and jerked me off my feet. Fortunately I got my ice axe anchored in. It was foggy, cloudy. Of course everything is flat light *then* so you can't really see anything. He just disappears and is pulling on the rope. Actually he fell off of a kind of cliff, he stepped off of one of these blocks or something and probably went down forty feet. So then we had to extract him out of that. He just walked. He couldn't see anything. It was all just flat light. And he just stepped off the edge of it and fell. Actually, he wasn't in a crevasse, so it was a little easier getting him out of there if I recall. It's kind of like being on a ten-story building downtown and you walk off the top of it accidently. I think we only really dropped somebody in a crevasse a couple times. Pretty lucky.

### McGonagall Pass

McGonagall Pass is where we get off the glacier—where we can take off the crampons and get rid of the snowshoes. And this is where we actually made a camp. Everybody's pretty tired because we've been walking for about 24 hours straight. And so we set up a camp. It was not really a nice day—a little damp. But everybody needed to rest a little bit here. We just tried to find a place between the rocks with your sleeping bag so we could lay down and get some sleep. Not a very comfortable campsite.

The McKinley River you want to try to cross early in the morning before the glaciers start melting up above. This river can come up a foot or two. If you're crossing it, that's enough water to make it dangerous. *In some places* it looks pretty placid. And it's braided, in other words there are several channels, usually three or four channels. So when you'd get across one, then you've got to cross another.

*Once you* get cross the river, there's a campground. That's where we were aiming for, because the park service had a bus starting at Wonder Lake the next morning that hauled hikers back out. We were anxious to make that bus—get out of there and get some good food. So we had about an eighty mile bus ride from Wonder Lake *to the train*, could be a little longer than that.

*The next morning* it wasn't raining and the weather was clear. So we had a lot of visibility which was nice. *Once we made it back to the train depot,* we sat and hung out and waited for the train. On the train we could to order a meal. And everybody ordered up a meal. As soon as it stopped and we got on the train, the first thing we did is get down the dining car and order hamburgers and French fries. So everybody ordered a meal and we gobbled that down. We talked Gary into letting us order two meals. So everybody ordered a second meal, didn't take long to scarf that down. *We could* see the weather was coming back in.

But we didn't really care at this point because we were inside and be warm. It's about a two hundred mile train ride, actually a little maybe a little more than that from McKinley Park to Anchorage. Wish I could tell you who all those people *I climbed with* were. But I've lost contact with them. They were a good bunch of people. And for the most part everybody got along well. At times you'd get kind of stressed out when something happens that you don't like going on — but anyway.

## Sanford and Drum

One of the peaks in the Wrangell St. Elias mountain range is Mount Sanford (16,237'). It's a volcanic peak that last erupted longer ago than I can remember. It's kind of a fun mountain to climb because if you do it on skis you can have this enormous downhill run when you go to come back. Probably the easiest way to climb this is to use Lynn Ellis the pilot out of Glennallen if he's still doing flying and fly up to the base of the peak, then use skins to finish off the climb.

When I did it several years ago there was geologist in University of Alaska - Fairbanks that was studying among other things, Mount Sanford. Mount Sanford has almost an 8,000' vertical face and it periodically peels snow, glaciers. Anyway he got hold of me and he found out we were going to climb it. What had happened is, about a year or so before this (or two) before the climb, people woke up one morning and saw this huge plume of they didn't know what it was — a volcano had erupted or what. There wasn't any noise particularly. But what it was was snow, glacial snow, peeling off the face. It fell straight down and when it hit the glacier at the bottom of the peak, it shot a bunch more snow and ice and people thought that the mountain erupted, but it hadn't.

Like I say this is a kind of a fun part of the mountain to climb. Mount Drum is kind of a twin to it. It's 12,000', a couple thousand lower than Mt. Sanford. We went into and climbed Mt. Drum. What did we do on that? I think we went in and used snowshoes because it was getting late in the season and we were concerned about the snow. But I would highly recommend flying, especially flying your packs and a couple of days' worth of food. Fly it up to the base of the mountain, start to climb there.

When we'd climb these peaks—two different times obviously, I suppose you could go down and climb one, and then descend, climb up the other one. And it's just a peak that takes about 5 to 7 days providing the weather is good. We were warned about the weather—weather coming up from Valdez area. You could be climbing on the peak in nothing but sunshine and shorts almost and then this enormous cloud or with big winds would come swooping around. Builds up on the back side of the mountain then comes sweeping around to the front side. And that's kind of unnerving especially if you're very far away from your tent trying to climb the peak. But we had pretty good luck with that too. I think we had a couple days on Sanford waiting out storms.

We had Lynn Ellis fly our gear in and we hiked in. And we had him actually, on one of the times, it was when we climbed Mount Sanford, we had an airdrop. But airdrops can go haywire in a hurry and I don't necessarily recommend them. I don't have much experience with them. We packed ours in Styrofoam and in a manner that everybody thought they would make it okay. They got out the door of the plane. They got out of that in fine shape. The problem was landing. Having the airdrop land was a little rough. We airlifted in a gallon of fuel. We thought we had it figured out, but we didn't. It pancaked in and that was it. We weren't going to use that for anything else.

We ended up like I say using Lynn Ellis to fly us in there. There was another guy that was going to fly us in, so I call him up from Anchorage the day before we were supposed to go, he said "Yeah, come on up." And so we loaded all the gear and drove to Glennallen and thought we'd be ready to fly out the next day.

He said "Well just go camp, you know, set your camp up. We're not quite ready to go yet. Set your camp up over there at the campground."

That guy, we could have all shot him. He ended up flying another group in ahead of us. And he just wasn't accommodating. Well he didn't do what he said he would do and that's fly us in. I mean, have to be a real dummy to think he wasn't doing it, I mean there's only one flight service, two flying in there. So I went down to the airstrip when we got back after that bit of news. I had used Lynn Ellis before that on a climb a few years before and he was real good. So I went down to ask him if he would fly us in there and he said "Sure, tomorrow." So that was great news.

Lynn Ellis is the epitome of the Alaska bush pilot. I won't say he takes chances, but he got my attention. What happened with us is there were four of us. It turns out there was a party of Japanese climbers just ahead of us. And they'd been there a week. They didn't know how to get hold of Lynn Ellis to fly them out, come back and get them. So after much discussion, one of the guys that was with me didn't speak Japanese but with hand signals, moans and groans, and things like that we were able to communicate enough with them to let them know that it was okay, our group would come in second and these guys would go in first. Or come out, I should be saying come out, because they'd been up there. Actually they'd been there a couple weeks already, getting low on food.

So anyway we got down to the last people up there to fly out, that'd be me. So the weather was deteriorating and I asked Lynn if it was still going to be okay to get out. And he said "Oh yeah, we'll get out. But it's going to get a little exciting. Probably."

To me, when I'm in a plane, I don't want anything exciting going on. I'll go to the airshow, but that's about as far as it goes. But anyway, Lynn told me, you know, he said "What we're gonna do... We're going to get to the back of this airstrip." And it's a bush airstrip — it's probably a couple hundred feet long if that. So he got the plane back, we got it pushed back there. And he said "What's gonna happen is... We're going to take off I'll get up to max speed and then when we hit that draw up there..."

Coming off the airstrip there was a draw. And so he said "But it'll be okay. And here's what's going to happen." He said "We're going to hit that draw, and the air currents are gonna be such that it's gonna lift us up. And we are going to end up kind of on the side of the plane, with the plane on its side. But it's okay."

And by golly, guess what? He was exactly right.

*We* got down to the end of that airstrip in the draw and we shot up in the air, and then went way up on the right side came all the way back down on the left. But he gained enough elevation that the plane would fly then. So I figured one of those trips a year was enough for me.

Well, there must be a hundred things I could say about this climb. Well actually there's not. It was pretty nondescript. On the second trip that I went in there on Tom Choate[23] went along. Tom is an old mountaineer from ten years before me. But Tom was a great guy to have on a trip. We'd climbed up to the peak that we were going to go to, made it to the summit. And that made us feel good, because there was a party of four or five other people from Anchorage that were attempting Drum but they got onto this ridge that kind of gets a little hairy. But we avoided that, we just climbed up and traversed a slope that's below this.

I mentioned Tom Choate and then I failed to say anything more about him. But anyway, Tom has a Ph.D. in ornithology or whatever the study of birds and little animals are. And so coming out, we were coming out, we did this climb in June. And the migration of the plover birds, I don't know if that's how you pronounce it, but anyway the little birds just cover that area up there with their eggs and hatch their eggs. And there were just hundreds of birds hanging out. And you could watch them. They would all play the broken wing trip. It was interesting. But anyway, Tom knew all the scientific things, what there was to know about these little birds and actually some of the bigger birds, and what was going on. It was more entertaining than when we climbed up. It just is a slug, especially if the weather is not particularly good.

So anyway, that's what I've got to say about these two peaks. They're very prominent from Glennallen—very prominent from anywhere along the highway. *They're* fun peaks—doable without a lot of climbing skills necessary. You can have the benefit *of hauling* your gear up to the mountain to the base with skins. If you climb it early enough in the year the snow should be right. And you can have a couple mile long run *on the way down.*

---

23    National Park Service, Denali National Park and Preserve, "Historical Timeline," NPS.gov, accessed December 11, 2013, http://www.nps.gov/dena/planyourvisit/climbinghistory.htm. Tim's friend Tom Choate's climbing days continue. The National Park Service notes that on June 28, 2013 he became the oldest man to summit Denali (Mount McKinley) at age 78.

# RACE DIRECTIONS

# MOUNTAIN RUNNING

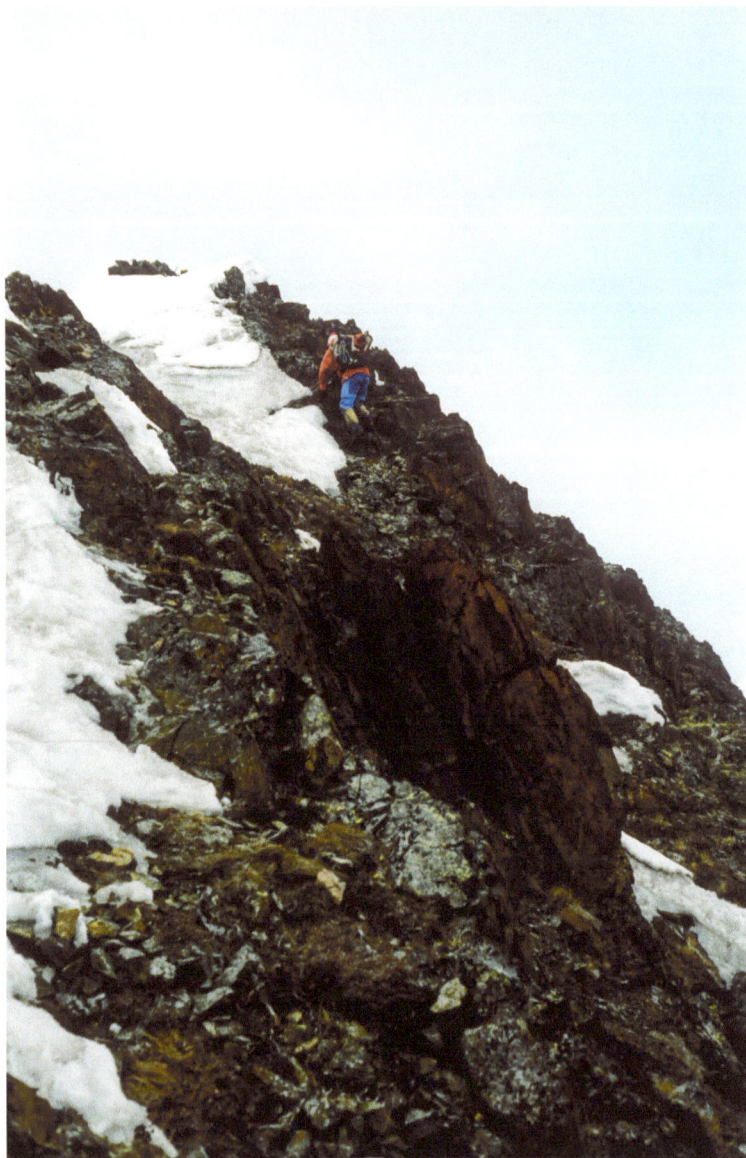

*Photo by Bonnie L. Campbell*

*Spring on Bird Ridge*

## Bird Ridge

There are two races that I put on, started. One of them is now the Robert Spurr Memorial Mountain Race and the other is the Crow Pass Race, called Crow Pass Crossing and many other things. I got a little concerned about some of the information that I was hearing about these two races. Doyle Woody from the Daily News called me up and had me give him a complete detail of how Crow Pass got started and when it got started, and more importantly, who started it and who was involved with it. But I will probably touch on that a little further down the road here. Right now I was going to talk about Bird Ridge.

Almost anybody that does any mountain running in Alaska, Anchorage uses Bird Ridge as kind of a training run. It's about the right height, almost 3,000'. About the right distance, something like a mile or two horizontal. And it's close to Anchorage, easy to get to, and a fairly safe run. The race actually started many years ago. When I originally started it, it was to be a summer solstice race. But it was pretty laid back and people were encouraged to bring a bottle or a glass of wine and cookies or something to celebrate the solstice with. So that's where the original name came from. And I believe in the first event there was about 5 to 10 people. We ran up. Actually we ran up Williwaw, we didn't run up Bird Ridge. So everybody celebrated the solstice and I don't remember much about it except that the weather wasn't bad and everybody that entered it had a gay old time. We didn't have things like awards or anything like that, but it was a good event.

Well a couple years passed and I decided to make Bird Ridge a little more formidable race. I knew Bill Spencer quite well and had talked to him about the prospects of doing that race, and he told me that many years ago—like me he doesn't remember anymore how many years ago—they did have a race from the Indian House or whatever bar that is closest to the base of the mountain. But I believe that was only run once maybe twice and that was it. So this time I just put the event in the runner's calendar. The problem was I couldn't get a permit.

The state park didn't want to have that become an event. So some people kind of fiercely fought it. And that was one thing that Crow Pass and Bird Ridge had in common. People concerned about the environment didn't like the idea of either of those races being run. And they had a point, however—like Bird Ridge—people are going do it unless you put a fence up around the whole place down there. Or you do what the Australians did on their high peaks and mountain runs. They put in steel matting. And you got to run on the matting. Now that's not really very esthetically pleasing. The only one good purpose is it saves the plant life in the surrounding area. Of course still people get off on the side, and run up the side. They don't stay on the trail and on and on.

So anyway, back to this. I got the race into the runner's calendar. Then I didn't advertise it. Actually only two people really knew anything about it—that was Nancy Pease and me. We decided to just keep it a secret, or not necessarily keep it a secret, but not tell people who was putting on the event. In the back of my mind I thought that this was probably only going to be a one race event, because the state park was going to chew me out regardless of what I did because I didn't get the permit. I didn't want to, I wasn't trying to defy them, but—they wanted to go through all kinds of hoops and environmental this and environmental that. That's all good, except that I didn't have time to try and get all that done and put the race on.

What we did was. I had a van. And I parked it at the base of the mountain. And Nancy was going to take over starting the gun, or shooting the starting gun and things like that. But the best of plans and the best of lousy plans go haywire and you have to kind of dig out from where you are and get it done. So the first race I put a wig on so nobody would know me and went down to the race. Didn't bother having a signup because at that time I figured the running community wasn't really big and everybody knew everybody else. So any one of us could make a list of who came in first, second, third, and fourth. Actually I did have results. I called up Doyle and gave them to him. To me it was an official race. However the next day, the state park folks had a long talk with me. They were going to issue Mr. Spencer a ticket for violating the permit law, whatever that is. But Bill really didn't know anything about it. So that wasn't fair to give him a ticket. So I told the park people that I did it. And I told them why I did it. I did it because I thought it was a good event. And people would be interested and it would promote the park a little bit more—regardless it didn't look good for us.

Well, the next year came around and the park folks kind of changed their mind and their attitude a little bit about what's a legitimate activity in the park and what isn't. Well everybody knows if you had a mountain bike race on that same course and you ran down to the finish line by running down the trail, which would be suicidal, but regardless, something like that and that kind of impact is going to cause erosion.

So anyway the next couple years the race got going. I'd advertise it. By then everybody knew where it was. And I had my first big crowd after about eight years. We broke 40 or 50 people in the race. Before that I had figured based on the number of people running Mount Marathon in Seward that we would get more than 45. So what I would do is go down to the Carr's store and buy cookies enough to feed twenty people or so and then bought some watermelon and that worked out real well.

Then it became popular. And it became popular very fast because Mount Marathon became popular very fast and kind of the thing to do. Since this was my race and I put it on. I also made sure that the race stopped on top. There was no racing down the hill. I could just envision the possible broken bones and skinned up bodies if we had turned around at the top and raced down. Also that leads to all kinds of problems when people cut corners, cutting the course, turning around two or three hundred yards before the actual turn around.

I'd go to the top *of the peak*. We had a ninety minute cutoff. And then I would turn around anybody who hadn't made it in ninety minutes and have them turn around and go back down. I always had a sweep, I always had two or three guys or gals, whatever, that would agree to follow the last runner down. So we knew where the last runner was and made sure the runner hadn't run off the course and gotten lost because it's possible to get lost on anything if you're tired and not thinking correctly.

I had some very good people come forward and say they'd help with the finish. The hardest thing I think that I had to do is try to figure out how to make a finish line record what was going on — what went on and the placings of the participants. I used this little unit that times and prints it on a piece of paper that the city had. Anyway, we tried to keep track of it that way, but the wind would be blowing. And it'd wind up the tape and we had a hell of a time. And then we'd have to start guessing where who placed. That got to be awkward.

I was really fortunate that my neighbor and friend, Kimball Forrest, agreed to take care of the signup and timing. And that was no small chore. As a matter of fact, Kimball—who was a good man with numbers and things—by the time I got down from the peak Kimball had the results. He was a real asset. Kathy and Laurie were two women that got involved and wanted to do the race, then I talked them into helping with the timing. So they along with people like Liz Butera helped at the finish line because the finish line could be pretty chaotic. To try to keep everybody separated so that we know who came in where *was challenging*. The bulk of the runners come in within ten, twelve minutes of the finish.

Through the years I've had a large number of people come up and help with the race. And like any event that somebody puts on—if you don't have the volunteers to help out, then you're not going to have an event. And it just always amazes me how many people show up and help and make the thing happen. The potential problem I had, especially early on with the race, was I would start the gun and I would climb up about a fourth of the way up the mountain and from there I could look down and see the race course. And that's where I'd start it from was up there I'd wave, wave something in the air. This also gave Jay Caldwell something to complain about because he was making fun of me standing up there waving my T-shirt to start the race. He said "Nobody does that."

I said "Well, I did."

But Jay did the race so I'll give him credit for that.

The other thing I did, and always liked to do with any race I was associated with, and that's make sure there was always somebody at the back of the race with a radio or some communication if somebody falls. Because people do fall and there are some places on the ridge where if you trip and fell you're probably going to get hurt and need some attention. Although fortunately we haven't had anybody really get seriously hurt.

The other thing is about putting on a race like this where you get up to the top and stop and turn around and go down, about fifty percent of the time the weather is so vile you can hardly stand it. You're lucky to stand up. It's raining, snowing. And we always encourage people to run with a wind shell or something to try to keep a little bit warm, but that never seems to work because people are hell bent to get as light as they can to the point of tearing off their number so they don't have to carry excess paper for their numbers. The other thing is it's a beautiful mountain and great scenery. So when you get up there you can stop, especially on the nice days and take a leisurely stroll down the mountain.

I think we used to have to try to get water up there, but that didn't always work. It was traditional to have watermelon and cookies. And the cookies came from Carr's[24] with their "10 cents-a-cookie" day. Then usually I'd tell them we're putting on a race and all that, they throw in a few more.

So the race grew and grew and then it became large enough where you had to put the brakes on it. So this was about the time when I was thinking that I was ready to retire, plus I needed to. I had some business dealings down in the "lower 48"[25] that needed my attention at least for a few days of the year. The only time to take care of this business was during the race. So I had to try to get somebody else to do it. And that wasn't hard. Bill Spencer took over and did a great job.

I don't think anybody should sit on something like this race for ten or twelve years, because—like when Bill took over for me, there were a lot of things he instantly improved on. One was the timing. That was could be a real potential headache. And everybody wants to know their time and they want to know it yesterday and not wait around for it. That was one thing about Kimball, by the time I got off the mountain with the sweep race of course being over, Kimball had all the results broken out. I was always impressed.

Incidentally, I changed the race name from the Summer Solstice Race a few years later after Bob Spurr had an accident and died on a mountain around Haines. To honor Bob, we made it the Robert Spurr

---

24    Carr's, "Our Story," Safeway, accessed December 16, 2013, http://www.carrsqc.com/ShopStores/Our-Story.page. Carr's is the main grocery store/supermarket chain in Anchorage.

25    Alaskans call the 48 states of the continental United States, the "lower 48." This includes all states except Alaska and Hawaii. Leaving Alaska is often referred to as going "Outside."

Memorial Mountain Race. And I figured I could do that. I'm the race director, why can't I?

So I can't think of too much else to talk about with this race. It was fun and I'm glad I had the opportunity to do it and glad that people came forward as they saw the race develop and volunteered to help out. I think it still is, maybe not a premiere event, but it's a good event. Good participation. People like it. Not too dangerous. And like I say, I don't know of many people that get hurt. The only person I know that got hurt on one of these races I put on is Nancy Pease. And Nancy and I were good old buddies. On the Crow Pass Crossing race one time she took a tumble and she probably got hurt worse than anybody else had. But she survived. Of course Nancy's a pretty tough character anyway, so that's no problem. This is about at the point where I'd like to, if this was handing out awards or something, I'd stand and say "Are there any questions?"

<chuckle>

"If there are none, then I'm going to go down and find myself a diet Pepsi and a donut. And indulge. Thank you."

## Crow Pass Crossing

The origins of the Crow Pass Crossing are from a kind of a hike, walk, run kind of activity that Bill Spencer, Jim Renkert, Nancy Pease and I did several years ago. It was from the parking lot at Crow Pass to the parking lot at the Eagle River Ranger Station. The four of us had been over that course probably several times. And this one particular day I just said "You know, this would be a good place to have a race." So we kind of had that in mind and semi-keeping track of our time. Although Jim Renkert carried a 35 mm camera was taking pictures along the way, the rest of us brought our lunch and had lunch. So it wasn't too serious. But the event took about, total time, just about six hours including a stop for lunch. When we got across Eagle River we stopped, wrung out our socks, and the total thing took five hours and something. Bill kept a running clock and that was about four hours. So in the end, when it was decided to make this thing a run, we put some limitations on the length of time people would have to do the event because I didn't want to have an event where people start at one end and go to the other end, but in between they go sight-seeing or take their camping gear or god knows what. It was to be a race, although not a serious race. *It was what* you would call a fun race — that's what this was supposed to be.

It ran into some snags when I went to get a permit from the state park and one from the National Park Service. Neither one of these agencies welcomed me with open arms with respect to putting on such an activity. Because supposedly in the wilderness areas, which part of Crow Pass is in a wilderness area, you're not supposed to have a competitive event. The other thing is, I had to come up with some kind of insurance to have insurance to run the race. And that became a problem. All the other things I was able to take care of—dealing with getting people to help along the way and just lining up volunteers to do different things and getting a course set. But the insurance was a problem.

So finally I went to my old friend Dr. Jay Caldwell. And he had an organization, a club you might say it was, called Old Folks Sports. And this, he had insurance for this. He told me that he would be more than happy to put his insurance on the Crow Pass race for me. And he also said he would be more than happy to volunteer because he thought that this would be a great thing. Now you have to understand Jay had never been anywhere on this course. And Jay was not a backcountry runner. However he has done Bird Ridge and he kind of looked forward to *assisting*. So we got the thing going. And not to drag this thing out forever, but anyway I got a permit for fifty people to run the race. And that was all. Fifty people. No more. No less.

So anyway, the day of the race the weather was, to put it mildly, very vile. Raining. Wind blowing the rain sideways. We had a pre-race meeting and I figured that probably half the people would show up that signed up. We were to show up at the parking lot about 8 o'clock in the morning up at Crow Pass. I thought well, if people drop out then we'll fill their spot with somebody because there was a wait list. The wait list people came down there and waited in the parking lot. All 52 that signed up showed up and there were an extra 10 or 15 people there. Before the race I decided *to let them run*. So I told Jay I was going to let these people run, but don't say anything to the park or the national *park*. If they provide an opportunity for you to say something, don't say anything about the number of people. Because I knew that I was violating their permit and they take these things rather seriously, which they should.

So off we go. The other thing is I had these cut-off times where it would cut-off if you didn't make it to the top of the pass *in time*. You had 90 minutes to make it. If you didn't make it, we'd have to turn you around, because there was the potential if someone took two or three hours to make it to the pass, then you had the potential problem of not being able to get down the other side in any kind of quick time. We didn't want to have to be out looking for people. So I got a sweep. A couple guys—one of them was in the race, Mark Kalinsky, and I asked him if he would volunteer to be a sweep. He really wanted to do the race, but he said if it would make a difference he would do it. I said "Well…" I had one other, Willy Hersman who was a sweep. He knew where the course went. That would be another problem. Make sure to get somebody that knows the route, because up in the pass it can get foggy. And this particular day it did get foggy. People got a little sidetracked. But I had brought this little electric lantern, *that* ran off batteries. So I took it up and put it on top of the actual pass. And it worked pretty good to guide people on along their way.

Well, I could see and I knew that this race had the potential to be pretty popular because it had a lot of things going for it. It was a good point-to-point race and it was very scenic. Glaciers, rivers, streams—matter of fact a couple years even had a bear or two in there. So there was a strong desire to have more than 52 people.

*When* we ran the first race Dr. Caldwell was supposed to get a couple of cases of Diet Pepsi or something and take it to the finish line. Well, *he* just looked at a map and saw how far it was from the start to finish and figured that he would make it in no time if he drove. However he didn't realize it was much shorter going the way we went—the way the race course goes. So *when* Dr. Caldwell got there, the top 4 or 5 people had already finished the race. But that's no problem. There were people there to fill in who came in what place.

I put the race on for four more years and, *as with Bird Ridge,* had developed some business in the lower forty-eight that I needed to attend to and the only time I could do it was in summer. So I asked Bill Spencer if he wanted to take over the race and Jay Caldwell said he wanted to take over the race. And I said "Well, somebody needs to take over the race." It needs to have an active race director but it should have somebody else. You know, a race shouldn't be put on the burden on one person's shoulders. They should get help from the people that run these races.

Anyway the race provided many opportunities to have some unusual things happen or go on. In one of them these people went across *that* were going to follow the racers. They camped out up on the pass, and that night they got excited because there was a bear wandering around their tent. So they blew the poor little bear away. And it was not a very big bear. But the biggest danger that I thought I could see happening is someone crossing the river and drowning, because that had happened before *on the river*. Eagle River is not an easy river. One time I was going to request or require that people go hand-in-hand, especially the people that are shorter *because* the water would be up to their chest. We strung a rope one year from one bank to the other, but that didn't really work out too well because the river started dragging on the rope. That became more dangerous than just wading in the river. People were supposed to come down the off the pass, come to the river, and then go up river. A half a mile up river, the river is braided out enough that its spread out and the current is not quite the problem. If you go down river, which is the way the old trail used to go years ago, then you get into channeled water — channeled river, which is about twice as deep and twice as fast as up river where it's braided. A couple years we told everybody — anybody that went downriver, we'd drop them from the race. *We were* going to be strict about this. It just had the potential of somebody drowning out there.

The other thing is getting volunteers to help. Getting them placed is a real chore with that race. The first couple years that I did it, we monitored the numbers — race numbers. At about four or five strategic points we would actually even stop *it* if there were two or three runners coming along to this checkpoint, we'd stop it for a couple of minutes if need be so we could record their number. *That way if* somebody didn't show up, we'd have an idea of what checkpoint they got to or didn't get to.

Anyway, the race has become more and more popular. The number of participants has grown to I can't remember what a good number would be. I go back to the numbers because the original race I had like 52, permit for 52, but as I was saying we let more than 52 *race*. We had 65 or something like that. Because everybody that signed up showed up and we had these extra people that were on standby that I could see really wanted to do this race. Since they probably got up at 4 in the morning to get ready, I thought well, what the heck. What could go wrong?

What went wrong was when the runners got to the other side and the news media was monitoring the race, Jay Caldwell said "oh and we ran, we had 65 participants" or something like that. So the park director didn't like that and let me know that he didn't like it. They were talking about giving me a ticket citing my lack of following the instructions that were on the permit. But we all survived that and it got to the point where the park and the national forest gave the race their blessings because it was a positive thing going on in the park. And environmentally it didn't do all that much damage. I mean, that river for one thing—one year it's on the east bank, next year it's on the west bank, flooding.

One year we had the hazard of bees, wasps, ground wasps. The first runner got across, second runner got across pretty well through the bee area. And as runners were coming across the section where the wasps were, the wasps were getting more and more irritated. And coming along the last few runners, some of them got several bee stings. Fortunately that really was kind of a one year deal. But we had a few people that got pretty well stung. But we had the medical people. We always had the medical people at the end of the race.

What's kind of interesting in talking to friends, I just kind of assume that everybody knows where Crow Pass is. But that's not so. There are a lot of people, especially new people to Alaska, they may have heard of Crow Pass for some reason. And some of them have read it in different publications that I believe have come out over the years *that* talk about Crow Pass races being one of the premiere races. It's been well run ever since it was started, but the scenery is so great. Some people have gone over Crow Pass during the race got to the other end turned around and walked back. And the distance is about twenty-five miles.

When I set the race course up and started it as a race, the media was very intent on having me put a distance *on it*. Was it twenty-six miles? Twenty-five miles? Twenty-four miles? My original intent was we'd keep track of the times and things and make it a race, but the real focus was to have a good Sunday afternoon run through your park and enjoy the scenery. Anyway the course is the old gold miner's course that allegedly went from Girdwood to Eagle River across the old Iditarod Trail. There seems to be some evidence that that actually in fact did happen because once you get up in the pass, especially if you're up there in a year where there's not snow six-feet-deep, you see remnants of the old mining equipment. And it's kind of a nice place to go on a picnic, go up and look at the mining stuff and climb around on the waterfalls. Not during the race of course. Just as a place to go recreate in the summertime. It has potential for avalanche so I wouldn't encourage anybody to go up along a trail that doesn't have some knowledge of avalanche potentials. If you think it looks like there could be an avalanche, then don't go.

I'll say one other thing that Dr. Caldwell wanted to do all the time was start the race down at Girdwood at the lodge and run up over the pass, but that would be long. It wouldn't add twice the distance but it would add another ten miles probably. And then there's always Dick Griffith, who runs around all over these mountains anyway. Now Dick is getting up there in years, but you'd never know it. He jogs fast, let me put it that way. He went one way and got down to the other end and had his beverage and food and turned around and walked back. It's about twenty-six miles. So that's about a fifty mile day. "Dick," I said "why are you going back?"

"Get my car."

Don't know whether he actually did leave his car back there, but I know he went back on the course.

And then there's Robert Spurr, who is the guy I named the Robert Spurr Memorial Mountain Race after. He would do the Crow Pass race and he was a real stickler for time. He wanted his time down to the second. And I said "Bob, we can't do that. We're not going to do that." Because we keep track of the time. But, you know, running the race is primary. Having an exact time, I know that people like to have exact time. And we get there within you know the hour — no, we get there within the minute now. But anyway Bob would call me up after the race and say "Next year, why don't you run the race backwards?"

I said "Bob, that would be two-thousand feet or more climbing." The Crow Pass area is in kind of a rain shadow. Bad weather can come and settle in there. Very, very seldom is there a period time when during the race it's not raining sideways or howling or snowing or something. So running the race backwards you're going up into this pass and that's where people get into trouble and have got into some serious trouble. The other thing is it would be harder to monitor. And people would be getting all their vertical elevation, or not all of it but most all of it, at the end of the race. So they'd have to run up two-thousand feet and it's not an easy run. It's not like running up and down Mount Marathon, but it still has its hazards.

I'm really happy that I had the opportunity to start this race and run it for a while and then have people continue it on. And it seems to be a race that will hold its own for a while. I don't think it will ever be, and it shouldn't be, a race that you'll have five hundred people in. I think the hundred and forty-two or whatever it was I finally settled on for a number to keep the parks happy is enough. Most years, there's a few people you've got to put on a standby list, but most of the time after the people have run the race once or twice that's good enough and they're ready to do something else. So the other thing is it's a race that has been a measure of a variety of people. Some of the best runners in Anchorage or in Alaska come down and have entered the race and run it and enjoyed it. Some people, like Kimball Forrest, have run it almost every year. But again, I'd just like to emphasize, that what makes this race and a lot of races, not a lot — _all_ races — go are people that volunteer. Crow Pass is kind of a commitment of time and energy. If you agree to be a sweep, then you're going to be trotting along behind the last runners. And all I can say about that is you get to enjoy the scenery more. And you can also probably — although I don't encourage it — take a sandwich. There's no place to stop. Once you start the race, you're somewhat committed. There's no sit down beside the trail and say "That's it, you want a ride out." There's no ride out. There's nothing in or out of there from the start of the race to the end of the race. And in between is, like I say it's twenty some miles of interesting terrain what not.

We've had several times the record will be broken by somebody that is not necessarily thought of as a mountain runner, but just a wanted to experience it and accepted the challenge. I'd love to give you some names on this, but my memory is fading from sight. And this is one of these times when my memory is failing me, because it's been going on for twenty some years—not my memory—but the race.

# ORIENTEERING

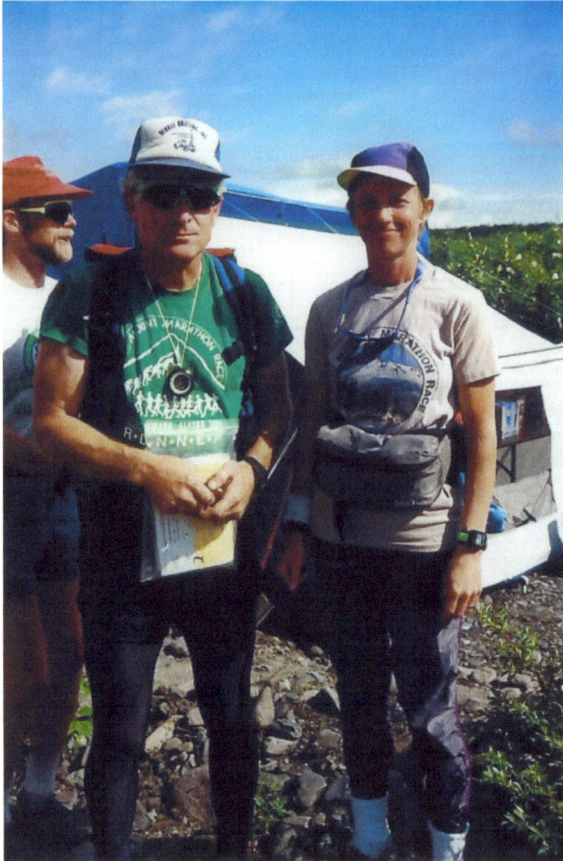

*Photo by Kyle Brown*

*Tim and Ellyn Brown (Jim Renkert background) at the Alaska Gold Strike Rogaine*

## Rogaine

*Over the years Tim enjoyed orienteering at various meets in Alaska. In the early 1990s the Arctic Orienteering Club held its first 24-hour orienteering races known as rogaines (Rough Outdoor Group Activity Involving Navigation and Endurance). Tim and Ellyn Brown teamed up for races in 1991 and 1992. Ellyn's articles replicated here and first published in Orienteering North America magazine, give a sense of these intense adventures.*

*In 1991, Tim and Ellyn competed in the Arctic Orienteering Club's first 24-hour Rogaine. Ellyn wrote the following article which appeared in the July 1992 issue of Orienteering North America magazine.*

## ALASKA GOLD STRIKE ROGAINE

*The Alaska Goldstrike Rogaine was held by Arctic OC on July 27–28, 1991. The Rogaine format is similar to a Score-O: you can take the controls in any order—but it is Score-O over a very wide area, most often using USGS maps. Teams of two or more have 8 or 24 hours to get the highest point total; usually points are deducted if your team arrives after the time limit.*

I didn't plan to take part in Alaska's first 24-hour Rogaine, because I expected houseguests then. But, as the event drew closer, I found it unbearable to think about missing it. When my friend Tim Neale called looking for a partner, I said, "You bet!" My guests and family could come along and camp with me the night prior to the Saturday morning start.

Getting to the Peters Hills, 90 miles north of Anchorage, took nearly four hours, because the last 37 miles was on a dirt road that deteriorated the farther we traveled on it. The pace gave ample opportunity to enjoy the spectacular scenery; the marshy meadows and spruce/birch forests we were driving through, and the two massive mountains looming above the foothills, 20,320' Mt. McKinley and the 17,400' Mt. Foraker. Both are located within Denali National Park, 40 miles to the north of the Peters Hills area of the Yentna Creek mining district.

About three miles from base camp we finally started climbing into some hills; the road cut into cliffs with dramatic drops on one side. Then one mile from the base camp, located at the junction of Peters Creek and Cottonwood Creek, was a bridge over Peters Creek that we were warned was closed. Though the bridge was missing a few boards, the race organizers had been driving over it—and they were comfortable enough, so we drove across too. We arrived at camp, after fording a couple of streams, when we found a sandbar that looked suitable for a good night's rest.

It was at this point I made my first tactical error: I should have stayed awake to see just when it got too dark to navigate with any efficiency. But, concerned with getting enough rest, I instead crawled into the tent about 11:30 p.m. while it was still light.

The Rogaine organizers, Arctic O-Club members Dan Ellsworth and Bill Spencer, selected this area after speaking with the local miners working claims in the area. The miners did not seem to mind a group of orienteers walking their land for 24 hours. A few even drove down to watch the start, scheduled to begin in traditional mining style with a blast of dynamite—but unfortunately the first was a dud. Although my partner and I were too far away to hear the dynamite that ended the 24-hour event, we were told the second blast did, in fact, occur.

This area, called the Yetna mining district, was first discovered in 1905. Over the years it has produced about 200,000 ounces of gold. The richest sections are at Cache and Peters Creek. Most of the gold is placer, however a few veins were located and also mined (placer: glacial or alluvial deposit of sand or gravel containing eroded particles of valuable minerals). Some coal deposits also exist in the area, and from approximately 1918 to the early 1920's, a large dredge in Cache Creek was powered by that coal. Today a few miners still work their claims. All we saw was a lot of gravel being moved around, en route to #33, and we saw very little mine workings anywhere else.

Saturday morning was again beautiful. We relaxed and watched the rest of the 52 people show up. But, I grew rather anxious as 10 a.m. drew close and still no sign of my partner. He finally showed up just in time; we got our maps and planned out strategy. The map covered about 50 square miles, with 55 stations that surrounded the base camp. The terrain was tree-less, alpine tundra-covered hills, rising from the base camp at 1800' to a maximum elevation of 4000'. The treeline in most of south central Alaska is about 1500'; so in this area the ridges are very walkable; in some of the lower areas and creek bottoms, thick stands of willows and alders make walking very difficult, but these could be avoided most of the time. Wildflower-laden slopes reach down from the ridges to marshy, flatter areas, dotted with numerous beaver ponds.

We were warned of bears beforehand, and advised to carry bear spray. It consists of a cayenne-filled canister that shoots a steady stream of cayenne into the face of the bear and scares them off. This strategy depends upon being accurate with an aerosol spray and not being downwind of the bear. I've been carrying the same can around with me for three years when I am in the backcountry alone, and I had no idea whether it would still work if I needed it — but I promised my partner that I would carry it for us.

The 55 control stations were numbered from the 20's through 100's; those in the 20's were worth 20 points, those in the 30's, 30 points, etc. The 100 pointers were farthest away from base camp, though often the easiest to spot. Dan and Bill set the course over a several-week period, locating the control sites initially from Dan's airplane, then relocating them on the ground. We were continually in awe of how much

work they had put in. They must have climbed nearly 20,000' and hiked 50 miles to get them all in. They attempted to make it impossible to get them all, a total of 2500 points.

Stations were set on the four separate ridges that surrounded the base camp, so we had planned to make three and optimistically four loops out of camp to get as many as possible. This way we wouldn't have to take too much food, because we could be back soon to replenish supplies. We chose to do the first loop on the ridge to the northwest of camp, as it was closes to Mt. Foraker and Mt. McKinley. They create their own climate, and rain, snow, or wind can come forth from that area any time. With good weather at the start, off we went.

Our feet got wet immediately — nothing really new to Orienteering in Alaska, and we got the first four stations readily, #26, #25, #45, and #35. We were instructed to sign in at every station and note our time and destination of our next station. This put an interesting aspect into the strategy, but for right now we were right behind Mike & Bob, a pair that we expected to do well. We wasted a lot of time looking for #29, and got a ways behind them at this point. The next five stations went well in spite of spending nearly an hour in a heavy downpour. I got quite chilled, and will take more warm clothes next year. Getting to #82 from #52 looked so easy—the same elevation; we thought we'd just walk on over there, but the side slope was very steep, and the footing difficult. We wished we'd climbed the extra 500' by staying on the ridge crest.

Where to go after #82 was the only disagreement Tim & I had about route selection. I (lazily) didn't want to drop 1000' to #61, then have to climb nearly back up again. I said we could get that one on the way back to camp, just an easy jaunt up a jeep trail. Fortunately, Tim agreed and we stayed high on the ridge to get the next three. What a view from #83, Mt. McKinley in all its grandeur, and even a view of the Tokositna Glacier, a 25-mile long glacier reaching to the south from Mt. Huntington. I wished I'd had a camera. On down to #65, #37, and #36, where we noticed that mike & Bob hadn't been to #36. So, they had decided to do the next ridge rather than heading back to camp. We studied the map again, decided we weren't all that tired, and had enough food to go on several more hours, so at 7:30 p.m. we headed east to do the northeast quadrant of the Rogaine.

So much for not being tired, after crossing the large Cottonwood Creek valley, we headed for #84, not even remotely thinking that we could make a mistake, but somehow we missed turning southwest in the valley, and ended up in the wrong cirque (cirque: a steep hollow, often containing a small lake, occurring at the upper end of some mountain valleys). Ooh, an 80-point mistake. We were rather mad at ourselves, finally deciding the map was incorrect at marking a prominent stream as coming out of the side cirque, when, in fact, it came out of the main cirque we blindly went up. Rather than go back and get it, we were high enough on the ridge that we went on to #32, #102, #43, and #49. About 10:30 p.m., after we both had taken pain relievers for our knees, we were 500' above #84; so upon dropping down and back up to get that, it was easy walking on to #38 and #66. It was getting difficult to see by 12:30 a.m.; we were tired, starting to get chilled again, thinking about how far behind Mike & Bob we were, when we heard Gunnar &

Jim singing, walking along the ridge towards us. They had already rested in camp after first doing the southeast quadrant, and were on their way to stay out all night up on this high ridge, then carry on, basically retracing our steps. I couldn't believe they were going to stay out all night. I thought they were crazy. They seemed in far too good a mood, in spite of saying they had trouble finding #63 and #39, and that they had no headlamps.

Because of the difficulty they had with those, we decided to get #57, then head back to camp for some rest. We couldn't see much of anything on the way to #56, we took a compass reading and walked, occasionally turning on Tim's headlamp when absolutely necessary (the batteries were weak), and luckily came right upon it. Now for the worst part of the whole Rogaine, the walk back to the camp through alders and willows, where we were warned by Bill and Dan that they had seen a sow with two cubs in this precise area—and it was dark. We yelled, sang, stumbled, praying not to stumble on a sleeping bear. We kept our eyes on the lights from the tents at camp off in the distance. Thank goodness for the lights.

At 2:30 a.m. we stumbled into camp, happy to find a huge pot of hot soup, bagels, and hot chocolate. While eating we got caught up on everyone else. All were in except Gunnar & Jim and the Tim & Tim Team. The latter team, also expected to do very well, had come in at 12:30 a.m. and were going out again at 3:30 a.m. In retrospect, that was the best time to take a rest, as those were the darkest hours. We crawled into bed, rested well, then up at 5 a.m. to continue.

The clouds were down at about the 2500' level as we headed for the southeast quadrant. I was tired, and it seemed to take forever to climb the 1500' to #58. Tim kept turning around to see if I was still coming. I felt I was holding him back. Once up on the ridge I was a bit better; we were trying to keep up with Ted & Pete, and Nancy & Wendy, both good teams. The clouds never lifted, navigating was very difficult, often we wandered with the two other teams, looking and looking for #86 and #59, the latter which we finally gave up on. Time was getting close, just before we got to #104. We ran into Mike & Bob, who were headed back into camp from 104, as they didn't feel they had time to get #103, so we were retracing their steps back to camp. This was about 10:30 a.m. We should have stopped at #104 and headed back, but when the other two teams caught us at 104, we all decided to look for #69 and #68. We wasted much time, and found nothing, so Tim and I finally left them still looking and headed back to camp, in spite of their warning that our choice to go straight down to the road via Slate Creek would be a mistake — Dan and Bill had said it was very brushy.

But, with tired legs, the thought of retracing our steps seemed to require to much vertical, so we went down. Cursing to ourselves all the way in the thick alders and willows. Looking at our watches as it neared 12 noon, we were bummed out, sure we had made a major error by going this way. The others were probably prancing along the treeless ridge and back in camp by now. Finally, about 12:05 p.m. we reached the road, and ran, yes, we ran, after hiking for nearly 22 hours, the nearly 6 miles on the road back to camp. As Tim tried to get me to pick up my pace, he asks, "Ellyn, got any water left?" I replied, "Sure, want some?" He briskly replies, "NO, dump it, Ellyn!"

To our amazement, we made it back before Nancy & Wendy and Ted & Pete. We were 17 minutes late, and they were 10 minutes behind us. Now, if we hadn't been 17 minutes late, which costs 10 points per minute, we would have had 1520 points, for 3rd place. Tardiness never pays; we had to settle for 1350 points, 6th place overall, but 1st in the Veteran Division and also the Mixed Division. This was good enough for a fine trophy made by Bill and Dan: a small vial of black sand with 7 or 8 gold flakes, mounted on a base plate with our names. The winners, Tim & Tim, were 1st with 2210 points and got a ½ ounce of gold flakes each; Mike & Bob were 2nd with 1630 points.

We learned a lot about Rogaining, but unfortunately, the rest of the competitors did too, so next year's will probably be just as competitive. It was way more fun than I expected, and the location and planning couldn't have been better, I can hardly wait until next summer.

The 1992 event is on July 25–26; contact: Ted Cahalane or Bryan Carey. (Remember, there's a 5-hour difference from the east coast!)

*In 1992, Tim and Ellyn again competed in the Arctic Orienteering Club's 24-hour Rogaine. Ellyn wrote the following article which appeared in the November 1992 issue of Orienteering North America magazine.*

## TANGLE LAKES ROGAINE

This year's Alaska Rogaine site was 270 miles northeast of Anchorage, just west of Paxson on the Denali Highway, in what is called the Tangle Lakes Area. Most of the Denali Highway is unpaved, although the base camp for the rogaine was just off a paved section of this seldom traveled road.

The Tangle Lakes are the result of the last ice age, during which the entire area was covered by ice. The higher areas are of volcanic rock, while the lower areas are glacially deposited landscapes of moraines dotted with numerous kettle lakes. The ice withdrew 10,000 years ago, after which stone age hunters spent time in the higher areas watching for game, leaving the area rich in archaeological treasures. Today the Bureau of Land Management manages the 55 square miles on which the rogaine was held. Ted Cahalane and Bryan Carey of the Arctic OC set up the course's 56 controls, and it amazed us how two people could have done this in two weekends-they really worked hard to make this a successful rogaine.

My partner Tim Neale and I thought we were prepared for this year's Alaska rogaine, having successfully completed last year's in a tie for 3rd, but the terrain was quite different from last year's. Although we covered 37 miles in 24 -hours again this year, we only scaled 13,000' of climb, compared to 27,000 last year. This year should have been easier on our knees, but unlike the higher and drier, often rocky terrain of last year's event this year's was more typical of much of Alaska, which is a world of spongy, mossy tundra. The alpine tundra consists of anywhere from 2 to 12 inches of low mat plants: moss, heath shrubs, dwarf herbs, bog blueberry, and bog cranberry. In the lower sections, the moist tundra consisted of dwarf shrubs, dwarf willows and alders and grass tussocks. These tussocks are tricky to negotiate, as you never know if a tussock will hold you up or bend with your weight to deposit you in the water. Both types of tundra act like sponges, holding more water than you can imagine, leaving no one with dry feet for the 24-hour period.

We camped the night before at the base camp along with most of the participants. The evening was beautiful, and we hoped for a great day ahead. At 5 a.m., however, the wind picked up, and soon it was raining hard, showing no signs of letting up. I crawled out of my tent at about 10 a.m., getting wet feet and chilling immediately. I was glad when Ted told us the start would be delayed for 2 hours. We expected Ron Rickman to emerge from his tent an unhappy camper, since his tent was now in a new stream bed, but he smiled as he stepped out into the water-his seamsealing job had worked well and all was dry inside.

With the delayed start, a few of us drove into Paxson to the lodge to get some breakfast, get warm, and stay out of the rain. I even got to eat breakfast with a good friend who was doing mineral exploration in the area, as she was waiting for repairs to her broken helicopter. She had been in the area a week and warned us of the numerous bears and wolves, but assured us that it would he

easy walking. Looking out at the pouring rain, I wondered why we were paying lo explore these hills and she was getting paid to explore them.

After a great breakfast, we headed back to camp, and by then it had quit raining, so the start would be shortly after 1:00 p.m. after all. We had ample time to get ready and plan a route, and as we all gathered for the start, Ted and Bryan expressed a wish to shorten the time to 23 hours, but some protested wanting to keep it at 24 hours. They reluctantly agreed, though they had a valid concern, since the later the event began, the less time they had to pick up the controls, and the fewer people would want to stay and help. Future 24-hour rogaines need to have more people involved in setting up and taking down the controls — the two Alaska events have taken a heavy toll on the two sets of organizers.

## OFF AND...
## RUNNING?

Off we went to 28, and by our second control at 33, our feet were soaked. We jogged down the road to 44, then across to 65, 76, and 33. The only tree and alder covered area was in crossing Clear Creek en route to 52, where we sang loudly to scare any bears away. We maintained a healthy pace, well aware of Mike Graham and Robert Tedrick on our heels. They were experienced Mountain runners and had placed 2nd in the first Alaska Rogaine in 1991. They caught us on the way to 56, on a route that was beautiful with wildflowers; monkshood, fireweed, and wild geraniums. Neither we nor they were really running—speed hiking was more like it—although on firmer downhills we often ran. We went on to 37, 73, and, finally on some solid rock, to 36. Mike and Robert were gaining 10 minutes a control on us. (Ed. Note: At each control, rogainers must log in their time of arrival and their next control destination. This is mainly for safety, but it allows later arrivals to see how far ahead others are.) We gave up trying to keep them in sight, wondering how they could go so fast. By now the sun was out, and it was really pleasant and beautiful. We jogged to 61 and 55, and en route to 82, we crossed paths With Kathy Sarns, Connie Hubbard, and Heather Moore. They said they had seen two grizzly bears, which had headed northeast up the valley, but were nowhere in sight now. Kathy and Connie were using the

rogaine as a training run for the 130 mile Ultimate Wilderness Run in a remote part of the Brooks Range 2 weeks later. From 82, the scenery was striking, a view of the Alaska Range to the north showing us Mt. Hayes at 13,832'. The last time we ran was from 26 down to 55, where Todd Shipley and Tammy Frankforter watched in amazement that anyone would be running. After easily walking to 46, 66, and 27, we met Anne Retherford and Lin Hinderman who had just come from 86. They were the last competitors we would encounter. This year Tim and I bypassed all the controls in the teens (worth 10 pts) and 20s (20 pts) we felt we had wasted time on those in 1991. We reached 75 by 11:30 p.m., only to find Bryan Carey waiting there with a camera. He filled us in on the progress of the others.

**ONWARD OR REST?**

This would have been a likely place for us to head back to camp for some rest, but my knee was beginning to hurt from the stress of the soft tundra, and I knew if I rested, I would not want to start up again. Though Tim and I had not talked about strategy, we both knew that we wanted, and needed, to stay out all night to be competitive with the top mountain runners that were out there. So we went on to 38 and 51, by which time it was getting rather dark. There was enough light lo get up to 39, but we actually had to search to see it once on top of the peak. At this latitude and time of year it does not get totally dark during any part of the night. There is always some light in the northern sky even when it is almost dark to the south. The darkest time is from 1:00 to 2:30 a.m., and we only used our headlamps to actually spot 68, occasionally en route to 84, and again to spot 84. We skipped 57, because, after hunting a long time for 84, we thought we would use up a lot of time hunting for 57, as it looked darker over there. The sky began to brighten as we approached 43, and brought with it enough warmth to raise a fine mist over the surface of the small lake there. It got even lighter on the way to 25, and we crossed the road at about 4:30 a.m., pressing on to 74. The lack of sleep caught up to us as we disagreed about the location of 41. A canyon appeared that really didn't show up on the map-it must have been just under 100 ft, so the 50 ft contour interval didn't do it justice. We crossed one too

many canyons, and as we came on the third one, we were looking at a dramatic narrow canyon filled with large lichen-covered boulders. As I imagined boulders cascading from both sides of the canyon. I prayed there would be no earthquake as we headed for 47.

My knee was aching by this time, and for someone who detests running on pavement, I found myself fantasizing about walking on nice firm pavement. I was glad for the easy walk to 64, 83, and back down to 45. As we headed down the valley toward 16 and 54, we could see that fog had developed close to the ground and was rising. Then a helicopter flew over; it was 9:00 a.m. and it was my geologist friend going to work. I envied her flying over all this tundra rather than walking. After our experience in 1991 of wasting time in heavy fog, we decided to get to 16 and 54 quickly, try for 85, and then head back to camp. My knee and the fog were not going to cause us to lose points by being late, as happened last year. Control 85 was not a problem, although crossing the river to head back to camp was. It was over waist deep in several places we tried, but we finally found a place that was only up to mid-thigh.

## THE FINISH IN SIGHT

Camp was visible uphill from the river, but between us and camp was a stand of willow several hundred yards wide, and it was raining. It is always trickier to walk uphill in willows, and after looking at our watches, toward 63, and toward camp, we decided to forget 63 and allow plenty of time to get back on time. It seemed to take forever, as my knee screamed every time I had to lift it over a willow branch. We had already talked about everything under the sun; I just moaned and Tim mumbled occasionally. I felt bad that my knee prevented us from getting 63, but felt relieved that it was almost over. Arriving in camp was more than relief-a folding chair never felt so comfortable, we got out of the weather, and had a great bowl of soup. Catching up on everyone else's experience was fun. Almost everyone stayed for the awards ceremony, held under a tarp between two cars.

As expected, Bill Spencer (one of 1991's organizers) and his partner Steve Bull placed first with 2350 points out of a possible 2500. Second again this year were Robert Tedrick and Mike Graham with 2280, followed by Dave Hart and Kristian Sieling with 1830, and then by Tim and me with 1800. We received a nice medal for first place in the Mixed Division as did the winners in the other divisions. Fortunately, no one encountered a bear, although when Bryan retrieved #23, he saw very fresh bear tracks in the area. Once again we learned that we should have taken more food—real food, like sandwiches. A common statement in post-nice discussions was "If I ever see another energy bar, I'll get sick!" It was fun to see so much new terrain. We had a great time, and we look forward to the next rogaine-now that we can look back at the Sogaine (spongy outdoor group activity involving navigation and endurance.)

# CROSS-COUNTRY SKIING

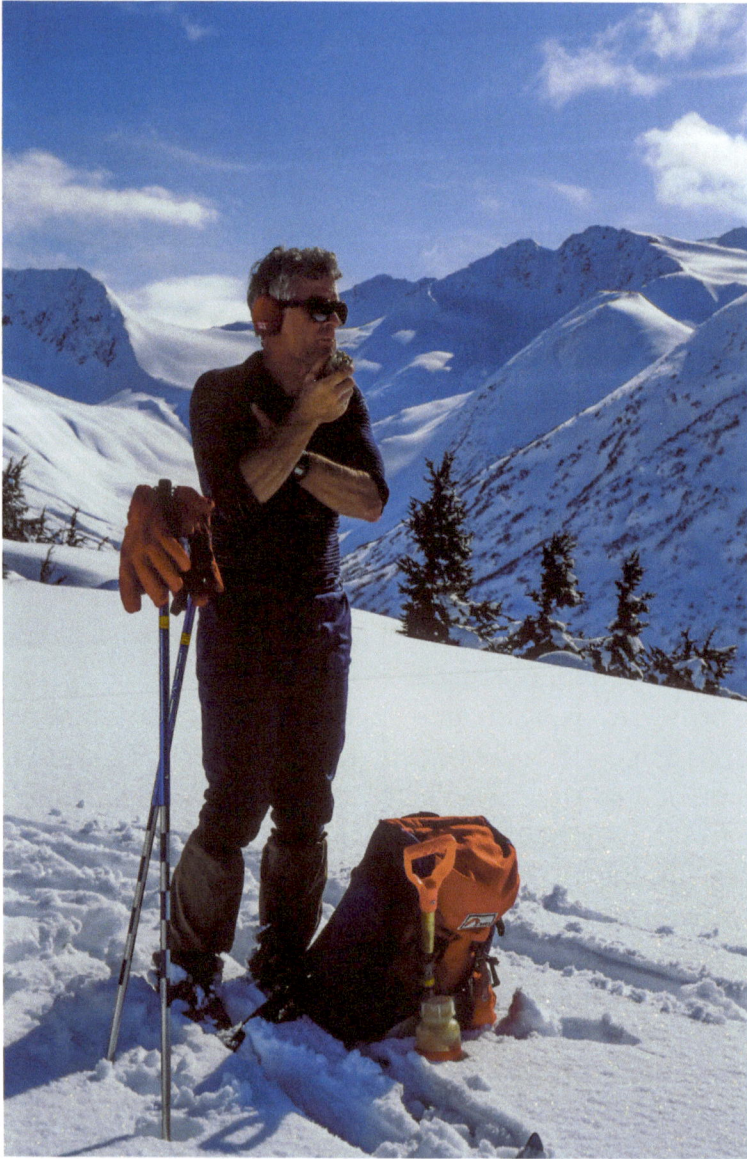

*Breaktime at Turnagain Pass*

Photo by Bonnie L. Campbell

## Race Director

One event that I was involved in, I was the race director for the World Masters Ski Race—cross country ski races in Anchorage. In March of 1992 Anchorage Alaska put on the 1992 World

Masters Nordic Ski Races. Basically out at Kincaid Park. This was a big event. Probably not the biggest event that Anchorage has sponsored, but it was a big one.

The style of skiing was beginning to change. It used to be all classical type, diagonal kind of stuff. One of the things that was somewhat significant about this particular race is they had the championship races and they used two disciplines—skate skiing and classic skiing. That was no big deal, except they were going to do them on the same day and on the same course. In the evening we set a classical course and then after those races were held, we'd take a break and take the grooming equipment and re-groom the course, let it set up as long as possible, and then use it as a skate ski course in the afternoon.

Well this hadn't been done. There was only one other race to my knowledge in Sweden the year before, couple years before, *where* they had put on some kind of a national race and had done the two different disciplines on the same course. So I called up the race director for Sweden and asked him about what pitfalls there were that it might be helpful for us to know so it would be fair for everybody, no matter what discipline you participated in. Of course, the ideal thing would probably be to use separate courses so you could set up a diagonal track on one course and use that the whole time. Not have to take the groomer and knock down the classical course. But anyway, we put it on and it did it.

So it ended up being a big event and there were over 500 people, all of them 50 and over—well, not all of them—but seniors. You could be a senior and be 38 years old. And it ended up being a pretty good event. We had a lot of participation from the volunteers who really make these races happen. I got involved in it because I had been a race director for a couple other big races and so they asked if I was interested in being race director for this. And I said "Not really" because I was supposedly going to go to Australia, well New Zealand actually, right around Christmas time. Around Easter time I got a call from a couple of people on the race committee for this World Masters and they asked if I would be the race director. And I said, well "I thought you already had a race director."

It turned out they actually didn't. The person that was going to be race director was a Swedish citizen and ultimately he could not get a permit to work for money on this venue. So *they* had to make some adjustments. Then they convinced me to do it. And I said "Well, I'll go ahead." I said "How much work has been done so far toward this event?"

"Well," they said "it was almost all done."

Well that's a perception that some people had, but other people didn't. One of the problems with putting this race on is this old thing of—you have five hundred and fifty participants and everybody has to have a number, an individual number. But they may have different numbers for different races. And you try to plan ahead of time as best you can to allocate *them*. Anyway you may have a group of skiers and there's fifty in that group, and another group there may be only ten participants at that. Say it's a 10k race. Well the men may be a certain number and then the women is another number, but for the same race. So you had to allocate those numbers, assign people a number. You had to know this ahead of time. And that wasn't easy. And if I didn't have Parkinson's now I'd be able to explain it better, but that's not going to happen. Oh, and then the other thing was, you had to have different markers for the different trails. These are all on little signboards you know like 12" x 12" or so. But there were some people helping me on that like Dick Mize. There were several other people but I just can't give their names right now. But there ended up I think I counted 200 volunteers that worked this race. If you didn't have the volunteers you wouldn't have this race. It's just that simple. Some of these people worked on the race were out there every day all day long.

We had some odd weather to say the least. First of all, a month before the race was to go on we were worrying about snow, and having enough snow to be able to put the race on. Well that ended up not happening. *Instead* we started to get too much snow. Short of having a snowstorm during the middle of a race and having it dump a foot of snow, usually too much snow is not a problem. But not enough snow especially on some of those courses like the Lekisch[26], where the biathlon range is, those corners up there in that—*on* those turns guys would come down

26   Nordic Skiing Association of Anchorage, "Trail History—Kincaid Park," accessed December 16, 2013, http://www.anchoragenordicski.com/

and slide around those corners, and there just wasn't enough snowpack on the trail to accommodate everybody sliding, doing a downhill type turn on the last couple of these corners. So they'd end up about halfway through the race they were ice. It was hard to make them work so that you didn't come down off those turns and hit a patch of ice. To do it right you'd need more snow up there and you'd need to make some snow, but that's a no-no in the Nordic ski world. Racing you can't, at that time, I don't know what it is today, but you couldn't put some rock salt up there *to* get some of that turn where it's kind of mushy snow.

Oh and one other thing about the weather, if I recall this correctly, which I think I am. The first couple days of the race it was cold. It was so cold that we, I think we ended up delaying a race one day or we delayed them a couple hours. And the thing to do was, I'd get a weather report from Dan who was taking care of the weather, the temperature. And so he would be on the coldest part of the course and we'd find out what that was, what the temperature was. And some of it was below minimums. It was over ten degrees minus Fahrenheit. But on other parts of the course, we had some parts of the course that were up there around ten degrees, twenty degrees Fahrenheit. So we had to do a little juggling there. But Dan was very adept at that and did an excellent job.

But the last race of the day, the last race of the series of the four, five days racing. Well it was a week of racing. On Sunday, I remember this, they held the 25k loppet—whatever it is. I can't even think of what that was anymore, but anyway. It got warm, and then we had some people start succumbing to the heat. They would dress too warm and then they would get down there along the coastal trail and no wind. Just ambient temperature is almost in the forties and people are overdressed. We ended up going down a few times to take the snow machine (toboggan) to go down to bring back a skier or two that had overheated and wasn't able to accommodate for it.

Anyway the race came off beautifully. Anchorage could have a gold medal for the effort they put into it, the equipment they have. They put on a first class race with probably a lot less people than a Sweden and Norway, some of these countries are fortunate to have. They're also

---

trails_history_kincaid.htm. Tim is referring to the trail constructed in memory of his friend Peter Lekisch's son Andrew Lekisch in Anchorage's Kinkaid Park.

countries that have five thousand, well not five thousand, but couple thousand spectators along the course. Anyway I said, after that race, I said "That's it for me for volunteering for race director. And I wish everybody good luck. I'm taking off for Australia. So I got out of there. Loaded up my bike and headed off to Australia for a couple months."

# BICYCLING

*Methow Valley Hill Climb*

Photo by Bonnie L. Campbell

## World Senior Games

When we did Mt. McKinley, we used snowshoes which are nice if you're walking, but they don't glide very well. Then I got into cross-country skiing and discovered what a joy that was. Then I was fooling around with climbing, hiking, skiing and that type of thing. Another natural thing to get involved in is bicycling. And I had bicycled actually more than I did any other sport. And as a matter of fact, when I was a kid in Spokane we had one of the city parks that I lived by. We would have bicycle races in the park. And it got pretty good. They were just kind of roundy round, similar to stock car racing. But they were a lot of fun. And they were semi-organized by my brother who had an affinity for being able to organize it and have fun. Like any racing, you want to know your results, and you want to know how far the race is and how long does it take ya to do the race. And who did you beat? Or who beat you?

Well I have done a lot of bicycle racing in a lot of good places and a lot of fun, fun races. But one of the best races that I did is in St.

George, Utah. It's called the World Senior Games for people fifty and older. During these senior games there are a lot of activities going on—different sports—there's softball, bowling, golf, tennis. Sports that seniors would involve themselves in. And it's usually over a two week period of time. And one week of it is dedicated to bicycle racing. They have mountain bike racing, but it's not quite as popular as road bike racing. The road race courses for the most part are excellent courses and a lot of fun. There are a couple hill climbs that are very interesting. There have been two guys in their nineties that would race. There were there every time I went there. And they would *do* the big hill climb they would do about half of that. But it still, it amazed me, how physically demanding the race is that these old gentlemen *raced*.

One thing about St. George is it can get hot. These races generally take place the first or second week of October. And it has done everything from snow on us to get around eighty or ninety degrees. So there's a variation of the temperature. So anybody who's going to go I would suggest you prepare for extremes. There generally are about two hundred people in these races. There's probably 15 women that participate. One advantage to going to St. George to race like this is you have some time in the evening. And before you race and after you race you can go down to Mesquite, Nevada and partake in the gambling.

St. George had a bit of notoriety back in the '40s and '50s actually, because the Atomic Energy Commission or whoever it is that handles the atomic bombs for the United States has set off a few of these things down there—underground bombs. They set them off just a few miles from St. George. That kind of made me nervous, but I asked some of the people that live there in St. George if it bothers them. They say—well it bothers them, but there's nothing they can do about it.

When I first started going down there now almost twenty-five years ago, there was a real presence of police. Sheriffs, state troopers, and the city police. Never at any time, especially in those early years, was there any mention of crime. Like getting your cars broken into or just getting mugged on the street or something. It's a real touristy town, but it's also well looked after by the police.

Some people go down there and do a few different events. Softball is real big. It's over, I think, over two or three thousand participants. Golf is very popular also because it's got—I don't know how many golf courses, but a lot of golf courses. The golfers tell me they're excellent courses—a lot of fun to play. And I mention all this because some participants in the bicycle racing also do some of the other events.

They had road bike racing and mountain bike racing. I only did the one because just dragging two bikes on the plane just got to be a hassle. And I enjoyed road bike racing.

For the road bike racers there are four events. A road race, a hill climb, a criterium—how many did I mention? Let's see if I can do this again? There's a road race, criterium, hill climb, and what's... Road race, hill climb, criterium...

Well anyway it'll come to me I hope. That's the problem with getting old I guess. A real problem with Parkinson's.

Anyway the road races are usually on a thirty to forty mile bike course. And it's interesting because a lot of these guys that enter these races, they've had a serious amount of road racing in their past. Some of them have been national champs. There are a couple of them that are actually even sponsored riders. But the criterium is in the downtown and it's a triangular course, but it's about probably a mile, maybe a little more than a mile around it. And boy, these guys showed me a thing or two about riding. They're fast into the corners, they're fast out of the corners. And if you're in their way they don't hesitate to bang. If I can remember right there are two, now I think they have three, but anyway there are two classes. It's like the amateurs and the beginners. And then you have the elite. The elite riders don't want beginners riding with them. And you can understand when you see how fast these guys go—especially in things like the criterium. The hill climb I could hold my own because I like hill climbing. And generally I do pretty well. The fourth race is the time trial and that's a twenty-five mile time trial. It's an out and back course through the farm country. And it's pretty. But you've got to be careful because the farmers don't care if you're out there racing or not. You don't get in their way or they'll run you over.

One thing about these World Senior Games is they put on a first class show. And actually they have an opening and closing ceremony that's pretty amazing. What they do is they draw all the Mormon kids into the auditorium where they sing and dance and put on a performance for the seniors. It's amazing because it seems like every Mormon kid is a musician or a good athlete. Well it figures, because they believe in hard work and they do *it*.

These games actually are incorporated. They have people in charge of the golf, the tennis, swimming, and bicycle racing. They hire this guy from California. I forget his name, but anyway he puts on bicycle racing, that's his job. He's got a pretty good sized trailer. In that thing he's got all the timing gear, course markers. He's also a race marshal, so if there's a dispute he or one of the people who works for him can mediate it. But it's just amazing. It's kind of like a mini-Olympic Trials game in the complexity of the way they put the thing on. But there's nothing you have to do as a rider except sign in and then get to the start line. Get yourself across the finish line before anybody else gets there.

The folks down there at St. George put on a really great race. I was extremely glad after I had done one or two of these races that I had been able to do any of them. Because in my plans, this period of time was beginning to get to the point where I was getting some itchy feet and wanted to not necessarily go out and bike race, but I just wanted to go do something with some adventure.

# DOWN UNDER

# BICYCLE TOURING

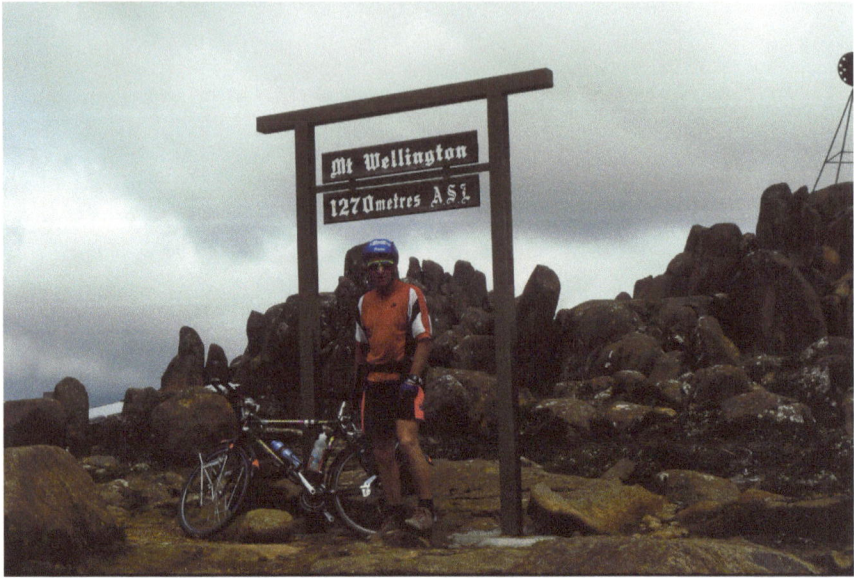

Photo courtesy Tim Neale

*Tim atop Mt Wellington*

## Australia by Bike

Well my adventures decided to take a slight turn and as I was on this one climb that we were gone about 3 almost 4 weeks. We spent most of my time stuck in a snow cave and looking for our food that was lost when a storm came in and buried everything. And I thought—geez, there must be a better way to spend my time not hung up in a snow cave for almost a month. So anyway, I looked around and thought, Australia. I always had wanted to go to Australia. And before I went in the army I looked into job possibilities that I could do working as an American citizen in Australia. Australia did have a program about that time where they would if you worked a year or two years at some job—it couldn't be just some menial task—but they would pay your transportation down and back. But I didn't get in on that.

So I finally talked to a couple of people that I knew that had been to Australia on a bicycle to see how plausible it was. And of course, they said "no problem." So anyway, I got my ticket, loaded up my mountain bike and flew down to Australia. I started in the north part up around

Captain Cook and continued to go north which is course going to a warmer and warmer and more tropical climate.

When I landed in Australia I had to make a diversion in my trip because I had intended to go into Sydney. But there was a problem *with* the plane and it ended up going into Brisbane. So anyway I loaded up my bike and took off going north, right into the tropics. Well, that was a mistake. I met up with this guy that was from Canada and he was doing what I was doing, but he was going to hang around this town for a few days and I wanted to get going. So I headed up towards Captain Cook. I got into this little town and there was a guy in there who had some sort of sign up that looked like he led tours or something. So he was kind of a guide so I signed up for his little tour. You know you go into the jungle in his boat. And he asked me how I was going to get around. And I told him on a bicycle. And then he said "Well, you know it rains a lot."

And I said "What's a lot?"

He said "Well, it can rain, you know, three feet in two days."

I didn't really believe him. But the next thing he told me made me a believer, he might have good suggestions. And one was. He asked "You know where to camp?"

I said "Well, I suppose. Are there campsites anywhere?"

"No, no. No campsites." he said. "But let me tell ya, don't just find an open spot by some river and decided to camp there because you're now in crocodile and alligator country. And they sometimes travel along the shore along these creeks looking for prospective food."

Anyway I got back from the little tour he had and I decided well, maybe I'll change my plans. So there I took off from this little town again and went the other direction. And it kind of started to rain. Now remember I just got into this country, so I wasn't familiar with weather patterns and what not. So it started to rain. And it rained quite a bit for about half hour, I thought well it's a cloudburst and it'll blow over. I was in a parking lot with about maybe 5–10 other cars and me on the bike. I went in to seek shelter in this little building. And when I came out I realized things had changed. What changed was the amount of water on the ground. There was just this sheet of water and it was about a foot or so deep *that* was flowing somewhat downhill. This caused me concern. So I thought well, I've got to get out of here. Then the next thing I knew, there was only one other vehicle in the parking lot. All of the other people vamoosed—got out of there, which is what I should have done. But I didn't do it.

There were some little native kids playing around where this road was, that was now buried under water. These little kids spoke English, but we had a little language barrier. They said, "We help you. We'll take your bike." So they hung onto my bike, I hung onto my bike. And this four-wheel drive thing that was the last vehicle in the area wouldn't stop and give me a ride. I was concerned about the wall of water, and how much water there was now. Water was getting up to my knees. And I thought—you know, this is not good. So we kept going and I got out to the other side. And I learned something that day. The paved road has dips in it, *and* a dip that may be a foot deep at its deepest point. So that's the way they had the bridges set up. Instead of the bridge going over the water of the stream, the bridges there where I was went down. So you went to a bridge, you went down. And a guy said the reason is they'd be losing bridges all the time if you had bridges that went over. And what you do is you wait till it stops raining and kind of drains off and go your merry way.

### Nolan

So anyway, I rode. Got on my bike and got going riding down the road. I heard my name being called. I thought who the hell knows me here. Well who it was, was Nolan Fontaine who was a Canadian citizen that worked the oil fields in Canada—a young guy probably in his late twenties. He had decided that he wanted to tour in Australia. So ultimately it ended up that he and I rode together for almost 1500 miles.

It was enjoyable to have a companion. I had toured before in Europe and other places. And I kind of had an idea how much stuff to take. If you're going to camp, you've got to have a tent and sleeping bag at least. And a little wad of spare clothes. The clothing was kind of optional almost because you're virtually wet all the time. So anyway, then you had to haul some food. Some places you had to haul water because the only water anywhere around was sure to be contaminated with giardia.

So I just got to the point of drinking a lot of Pepsi and Coke and water. Spring water.

So anyway Nolan Fontaine and I rode together for a thousand miles. He got off the plane and we went to baggage and we met up or saw each other again and had a talk. Then that's when he asked me which way I was going and where. I told him. And it wasn't exactly what he had intended to do, so we kind of parted ways. That's when I went north trying to go to Captain Cook and he went the other direction. So I thought well, that's the last I'll ever see of Nolan. But when I came back, I stayed up a couple days on this road that I rode up where all the water was. It was beautiful country. As long as I stayed near some running water they said that crocs won't get you. Anyway, here I am riding out of town and I hear my name, somebody yelling my name. And I thought now who would know me? It was Nolan.

He said "Hey you got anybody? You want me to ride with ya?"

And I said "Well, if you want to you can. Basically, here's where I'm going if you want to go, fine."

The other notable thing that I realized about this is Nolan had taken his bike to the post office and stripped off about fifty percent of his gear that he had in his panniers. When he started out from Edmonton he had tent, sleeping bag, pad, cooking stuff, you name it he had it. He got to Australia and after about two or three days, he jettisoned his sleeping bag, his tent, his stove, just about everything. Decided it was all going to be too heavy. But one thing he wouldn't get rid of was his boombox.

So he kind of went from the extreme of having everything but the kitchen sink to having virtually nothing but his shorts, T-shirt, and this boombox that he had tied to this back rack on his bike. Well eventually Nolan realized that he needed a sleeping bag, or more than anything he needed a tent. And I had cooking gear so we didn't worry about that. But Nolan and his boombox—he liked his music. He had it rigged up so that he could reach back and change the tape or whatever. And there we would be—the two of us riding down the road on our bikes.

Now we didn't run into many people. I think in the little over 1200 miles I think we saw four people. It was either two or four people. And we realized why. Because when Nolan went into a barbershop got his haircut and gets talking to the woman giving the haircut she told him "You're crazy if you ride a bike up here." She said that her friend or relative or somebody was just killed the last week on a bike. The problem is there's no shoulder. There's pavement and a line, but no shoulder. But at least we had mountain bikes and not road bikes trying to deal with all the garbage in the road.

But Nolan eventually acquired his tent. I think he also got some kind of a sleeping bag. It was a great time riding with Nolan. We'd be approaching this little town or something and you could hear this boombox probably ten miles away it seemed like. When he came through town, you don't see some guy carrying a boombox around full volume very often. But there was Nolan. He was doing it. People were coming out to see what the racket was. We were kind of a spectacle. Normally I don't like to draw attention to myself traveling like that. But it was okay, it was nice to have music to listen to.

Eventually Nolan and I parted ways. He went to Brisbane or Sidney, I don't remember which. He was going to hang out with some friends of his that lived there from Calgary. So he told me when we parted company –this was the day of no cell phones—if I was to mail something to somebody across Australia it would take a few days to get there at best. So anyway, sadly we parted company. We parted friends which is good. And I kind of missed his boombox after he was gone. Nolan.

When I got home there was a letter from Nolan. He had sent me from Australia, but he couldn't send it to me *there*. It went to my address in Anchorage. He knew I was heading south eventually towards Melbourne and he was going to stay with these people. What happened was he ended up staying there a couple of days and realized that was a mistake. The people had said come on you can spend some time with us. But in fact they probably didn't expect for him to really show up. So he realized he wasn't real welcome. So he decided to take off and try to catch me. But he happened to leave me at a point where I was ready to get in some 60, 70, 80 mile days instead of wallowing around in 25 or 50 miles. And Nolan just had to guess which road I'd take, but there weren't many roads. There was essentially one road up and down the coast of Australia there, the main road. I say main road, because that's where all the trucks, the tour buses, the people, the wackos and nuts, everybody gets out there. They're either driving ninety miles an hour or else they're running you off the road.

A little sidebar here. When I was up north and riding up at Camp Cook, I discovered that there was a dirt road that had eight feet, seven feet on either side of this paved strip. So cars going one direction would hang both sides off the asphalt and then when they'd pass. They would both share the road. So it was either being shared or used. And I looked at this, watching this I thought, I should do this because I'd rather ride on the pavement too. So, I thought well give it a try. That almost became a fatal mistake because the Australians decided not give way to a bicycle. They don't count. And I have to say, Australia is a great place to ride to a degree and a great country, but boy-oh-boy the drivers. They don't like you, don't like you on their road.

## Hostel or Hostile?

When I was traveling around Australia on my bicycle I found it convenient to spend the night at a backpacker's hostel sometimes. They're different than the youth hostel in that the backpackers are designed really more for transient people—especially transient field workers picking fruit and what not. And they don't have many restrictions. They allow alcohol in the places. They're pretty cheap though. So anyway one night I decided, I can't remember why, I don't even know if I thought about it. But anyway I decided to stay in a backpackers. I was a member of the American Youth Hostel Association, but sometimes it gets to be a hassle trying to stay there and then they have a lot of restrictions on you. So anyway, this one night I thought just convenient to stay in the backpackers for a break from sleeping in the tent, fighting off bugs.

So I got in this place and there were about probably six, eight guys already there. They were field workers that had gotten off *work*, got their Foster beer and were having a good old time in the kitchen. Well they were pretty noisy and I was really tired. I was trying to ride a couple consecutive days of a hundred miles to see if I could do it. So, about midnight, or god knows what time it was, these guys in the hostel had got pretty loud. A lot of yelling and I couldn't get any sleep. There were a couple of other people in the hostel the same as me trying to get some sleep. So I just said geez I've got to see if these guys will quiet down. So I walked down there to their room, or actually they were in the kitchen. I asked them if they would mind please quieting down a little bit so we could sleep, the rest of us. I discovered that that was a mistake because a couple of these guys got pretty excited. Probably had something to do with the fact that I was an American and not an Australian or New Zealander. So this guy decides he's going to pick a fight with me and pulls out this knife. Starts weaving, waving it around and I figure it's time to get out of here. So finally I did get him off of me and away from me. I picked up a chair with four legs, like a kitchen chair, and shoved him up against the wall. Then actually a couple guys came in and helped me. We got the knife away from the guy and I don't know what else happened. It was probably early, early in the morning when things calmed down. But I decided I don't think I'm going to go in and tell a group of guys to be quiet. *<laughs>* Especially when they've been drinking.

### Boombox

When I would be riding along down the highway and come to a little town, I'd pull into the little town. The main road went right through town so you didn't have any choice but to go through town. And a lot of times there'd be one or two bars in these towns. And in Australia for whatever reason they leave the windows open. It's more like a shutter that goes over the window. And when I came riding into town It breaks up their day. The locals that live there, they'd come out and start asking me a hundred million questions.

When I was riding with my friend Nolan he had this boombox on the back of his bike. So as we were coming down the highway, and there's only the sheep and cattle out there along the road. People would hear us coming for about a mile away I swear. Of course that brought more people outside to see what on earth is making all this noise? And it would be Nolan. But he's a jovial character and I think it amused people to no end to see something like that.

### English Translation

It's funny how we speak the same language as Australians and New Zealanders, but some of the words mean things *that are* completely different. It's like get in the line and cue up. Is that even it, I think that's it — cue up.

And one of the big ones I got embarrassed by, when I would be riding around or something I'd stop at a little restaurant and get something off the barbie and my hand's would be greasy. So I'd just take a napkin type thing and wipe my hands. I was just in the habit of kind of if I ordered some food, especially something greasy I'd ask if I could have a napkin please. People would snicker and laugh. And I thought "what is all of this all about?" So finally I was in this little store, or little restaurant, and I asked for a napkin..

The woman said "You're an American."

And I said "Yeah, how do you know that?"

She said "Well, I have to tell you something. In Australia, a napkin is something a woman would use at certain times of the month. And it's not something to wipe your food off your hands."

"So you mean I've been driving around in here for a month almost and been asking for napkins and nobody said anything to me?"

She just laughed. "That's why I'm telling you now."

### Australian Roads

Another thing that I discovered was probably a misconception about Australia. And that's everybody finds the Australians so friendly and nice and helpful and all that. And that's true. Until they get in their car. When they get in their car they don't have much use for bicycles and bicycle riders. There are times when I would see as I got closer to Sydney and I saw bicyclists out on the road. They would ride two and three abreast and create a mini-traffic jam and create a bunch of pissed off people driving down the road and honking their horns. So I decided there are friendly people, but don't push it — especially if you're on a bicycle.

I learned that most of the Australian roads just had the main road which was two lanes, one in each direction, but no side road. The side of the road — the shoulder — doesn't exist. It's about two inches wide if that. So it took a while to kind of get used to that plus driving on the wrong side of the road.

### Sheep

The times that I've been in Australia on my bike, I think I've been down there three times; I try to make it to Tasmania. It's like an island and it's a lot more bicycle friendly. And it's a nice bike ride. Just going from west to east or east to west, you get into about three climatic, temperature climates. You get semi-tropical and lots of rain, pretty arid and almost a desert. You *also* got the usual animals around there bouncing around. Kind of interesting.

When I was riding my bike down in Tasmania I saw a herd of sheep coming up the road like when I would herd the sheep up to Browning, Montana. This band of sheep was taking up the whole road so I had nothing to do but wait for them. They were on a bridge. The usual thing when sheep are on a bridge. They stand there and "baa-aaa baa—aaa baa—aaa."

So anyway I'm at the back of this pack, or at the front of it I guess you'd say. I look up and the sheepherder was this woman. And I tell you what. There are some beautiful women in Australia. And this was one of them. Herding sheep.

### Velodrome

Australians are good bicycle riders and good bicycle racers. Usually I think they gather up a few Olympic metals every time the Olympics come along. In Tasmania they have what they call a velodrome. I think they call it a velodrome. It's a wooden track, it's not very long, about an eighth of a mile maybe a little bit less. A circle, and again it's wood. On the bottom on the track, it's flat. When you get all the way to the top of the track it's almost 90 degrees. You can't stay there if you're just sitting. You'd fall off.

But they do this motor paced racing. This would be a great thing for Anchorage if they built a track like that and held races, because it's a great spectator sport. You can see the whole track. Basically there's a lead vehicle and it starts going around the track and it gets up to about five or six or maybe seven laps. They're short. They're going "wheee, wheee, wheee." Then when it's motor paced, they'll have a motorcycle out front. When they really get serious they have a motorcycle out front and they have like a piece of plywood on the front of the motorcycle to create a *draft*. You know, so that the guys behind don't have this wind they're fighting. And they can get up to almost fifty miles an hour. But it's not done very many places. I think the only place I know of in the Northwest that has a velodrome track is Marymoor, out of Seattle. But it's pretty exciting stuff. And it's just these super sprints.

Another thing is, they don't have brakes. Actually what they have is two gears. They have a cog on the back and they have a gear on the front. And then they just start pedaling. Somebody will lead out. Break away from the pack and try to get away. They've got to really be in shape. All these people that do this, not motor paced, but also the other type of closed circuit racing like this; everybody that does that — women and men — have these super muscular thighs because it's just an all-out sprint, each race you're in. You may have to go for half a lap, but it's pretty exciting.

## New Zealand

One trip I made it was a relatively short little adventure I think it was only about a month long. But it was actually right after the World Senior Games in Nordic skiing back in 1992. I took off for New Zealand. I was going to tour around New Zealand with a friend who ended up being my personal guide, which was really nice. She also helped us get bicycles to be able to be able to ride for a little while. I ended up renting a car with the help of my friend. It was easier getting around than hitchhiking or taking the train or the bus.

ALASKA

# ALASKAN ADVENTURES

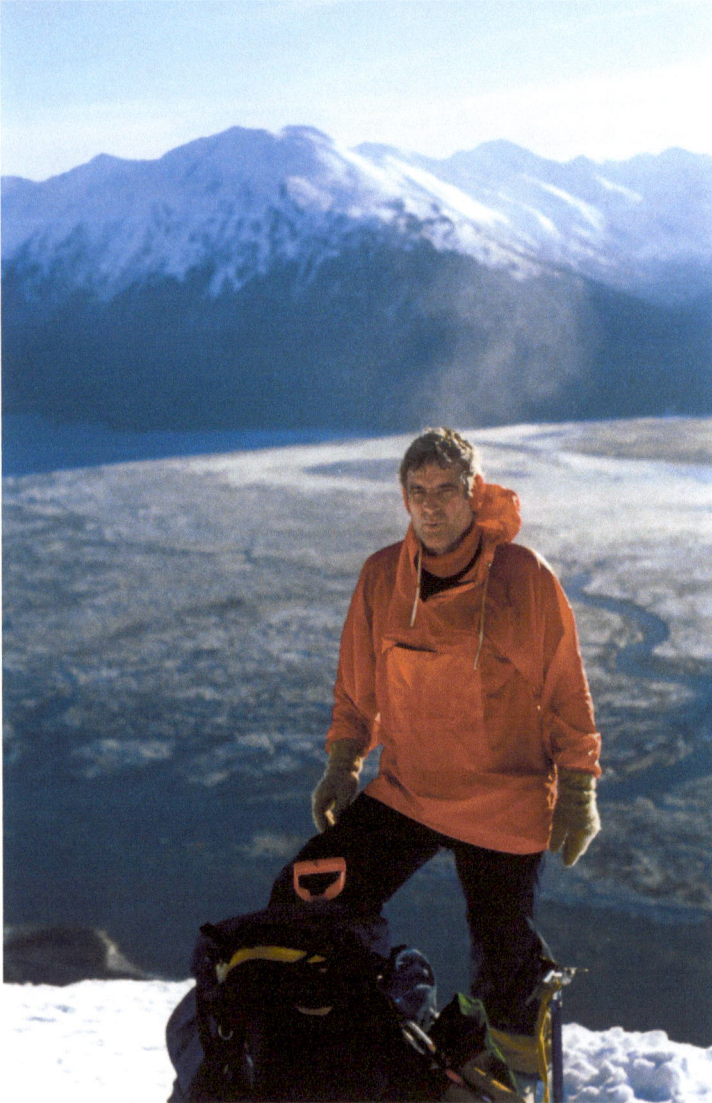

Photo by Bonnie L. Campbell

*Winter Climbing in the Chugach above Turnagain Arm*

## Cold!

One winter, between Thanksgiving and Christmas or New Years I flew down to Seattle and spent Christmas down there. A lady I worked with in Anchorage had promised a friend of hers that she would bring this friend's car back to Anchorage from Seattle. She didn't want to drive alone, so she asked if I would go with her. So I said "Yeah. What are we going to drive back?" It was a little pickup, little Datsun or Toyota or something, little pickup. And I said "Well, has it been winterized?"

She said "Yeah." She talked to her friend and her friend said that her dad took it down to a service station in Seattle and had it winterized. Well, I should have been a little more careful about that statement as to how much of it was not exactly accurate. Not that anybody was trying to mislead anybody. But anyway we started out from Seattle one fine afternoon and figured that this should be a relatively uneventful activity. And it kind of was. Our clue that we might be in for a little bit of a surprise was when we got up to northern Washington, can't even think of the name of the town up there that you go across the border. It was snowing, which isn't exactly unusual, but it was just a little early. But the weather was cold, *and* getting colder. So we got up and crossed the Canadian border. Can't even think of the name of the first town we got to, but anyway.

It was cold. It was beginning to get maybe around ten degrees, something like that. So we got into Canada up about a hundred miles north of the border, decided to stay in a motel there *and* take off the next day. Well the car wouldn't start—that was a bad sign. So we ended up needing to get the car jump-started. Then we went up to Dawson Creek, that's about 300 miles north of the US-Canadian border[27]. I opened up the hood to just check, you know, just check the engine. The liquid in the radiator was just slush. That's really not good at all. We've got to do something. So I told her we had to get some antifreeze or do something. But if it's slush at twenty degrees, here it's going to be ice when we get up another hundred miles or so. So I took the car to a service station, *and* the guy wasn't going to change the antifreeze for me. He wasn't going to do anything actually. I can't remember what the deal was, but he said that he'd sell me some more antifreeze and *that* I'd want *to* put it in myself. So that's what I did.

---

27    Google, "Blaine, WA to Dawson Creek, BC," *Google Maps*, accessed June 26, 2013, https://maps.google.com. Google Maps shows the main border crossing into British Columbia is in Blaine, WA which is about 720 miles south of Dawson Creek, BC.

Then we got up to Watson Lake. And we had a problem there because the car wouldn't start again. Now it was getting cold. Now we're talking about minus five, minus ten. So we ended up there was another car there, another couple, a family that was going to the Kenai or some place. And they were at Watson Lake. Neither of us could get our cars started. So his car was better, almost starting. So we took the battery out of *our* car. We paid twenty-five dollars or something like that, and this guy put a weed blower — a weed burner — under the car for five minutes or something like that. Anyway we got her car started. And then I switched the batteries around. So our battery was charged.

When I took the battery out of our car, I took it into the lodge and stuck it behind the chair. But I didn't tell the lodge owner, because I figured he probably would have charged me another twenty-five dollars. He had a wrecker that was in this garage. He was just keeping it in there, but he didn't want to bring it out. He would jump start us, but that would cost an ungodly amount of money anyway. To make a long story short, we got this guy's car started then eventually we got *our* car started and decided to head out for Anchorage. So we traveled together for a while. We got up into northern Yukon. He wanted to stay overnight and my friend wanted to go. She just wanted to get out of there and go. So we took off. We got up to Tok. It was cold — matter of fact we could barely see out the window because the defroster couldn't keep up with the ice. So we got into Tok and I saw these guys that I knew. They were running some drills — soil testing equipment. And they said that they were shutting everything down because they couldn't keep up. It was too cold. Thermometer said sixty-five below zero. Hard to say exactly how cold it actually was. But I'm sure it wasn't colder. But it could have been minus sixty-two very reasonably. And so here we were trying to make up our mind what to do. We decided if we stayed there overnight that we'd have to do something major to get the car started in the morning. It just wasn't going to do it. So we decided to keep the car running. And then we heard that the temperature in Glennallen was like minus twenty or something which was like a heat wave for us. So we figured, well we get to Glennallen we should be able to make it to Anchorage without too much of a problem. That's what we thought anyway. So we take off out of Tok. And from Tok to Glennallen there's not much of anything. There's little Mentasta Lodge and Slana. I knew a guy that worked for the state at Slana and I figured if we had a breakdown we'd have to get there. Now Renee and I were wearing all of our clothes to stay warm. I had thrown a pair of insulated coveralls in the car. And between the two of us we came up with enough clothes to keep us warm while we were in the car it was running.

Up at Tok, we had something to eat. Just left the car running and got in the car and took off. We drive down about sixty miles. Nothing and nobody around anywhere. Driving along and the car just quits. One minute its running and the next minute it's not. So here we are probably sixty miles from anywhere and I said "Well Renee, we've got one chance probably to get this car started. We'll take that right now before it cools down any more than it is."

So I started the car and—yahoo!—it started. We never stopped or slowed down the rest of the way. We got to Glennallen and it was slightly warmer and we could get out. Didn't stop the car, but we could get out of the car and walk around. The windshield was beginning to defrost a little bit. But anyway I found out later what more than likely happened and that's the carburetor can ice up. Normally on the carburetor there's some little heat vents that come off of the manifold and go up to the carburetor to keep it slightly warm, almost hot. But when it's sixty-five or sixty below zero that little heat manifold isn't enough to keep the car from icing up..

This is the problem *for* pilots years ago—before they knew about icing carburetors. They'd take off, and they'd fly. They were doing what we were doing. And then they'd crash. Kill everybody on board whoever that was. And they didn't know why. They'd take the plane apart and there was absolutely nothing wrong. Had fuel. But they finally discovered this icing problem. The carburetor on the airplane engines succumbed to this icing problem. We were lucky because we weren't flying of course. But it didn't take long for that carburetor to, you know, get heat off the manifold and it probably would have lasted ten minutes or so. But when it restarted we were very fortunate. And that's probably about the coldest weather that I have ever experienced. When I worked in Prudhoe Bay they talk about the windchill—now that gets cold. But the ambient temperature doesn't get as cold as Tok and some of those places. They get seriously cold. And I only had one other experience with being out driving someplace when it's that cold.

## Fortymile

Well one particularly fine fall day a few years ago. A friend of mine and I were sitting around thinking how can we take advantage of this great weather? This friend was actually a good canoe person, and could navigate and use a canoe pretty well. So the two of us decided to load the pickup up with the canoe and up we go to the Fortymile river. The idea was to float down the Fortymile at O'Brien Creek and float into the Yukon River and then float down the Yukon River to Eagle, Alaska. That's the way it sounded and that's the way it started out. So we shoved off. One thing about this I should mention, once you push off into the river you can't get out till you get down to Fortymile. We figured that wouldn't be a problem.

So we got up to the Fortymile and unloaded the canoe, got it to where we could come back and get it. And we pushed off and away we went. We started kind of late, so we decided just to go a little ways. So we went about six miles and we found a place to camp. It was actually a trapper cabin, miner's cabin or something. It was in disrepair, but at least it was something over our head. Actually it had an old wood stove in there and we could heat that up because it snowed.  It snowed about six inches—so much for the good weather report.

So the next day we were floating down the river and we come upon this pile of debris, logs, branches, you know just all kinds of stuff. Obviously, there had been a flood upriver at some point. Couldn't tell whether it had been this year, last year, or when it was exactly. We come scooting by this thing and I said "Whoa, wait a minute here. Pull over"

So we pull over. And there in the pile of junk, debris, and garbage looked like a dredge. So we drug it out of the pile of debris and thought—well, we could either take it back to Eagle and get it to the rightful owner, or who knows what. So we put the thing in the middle of the canoe. We didn't see that that was a mistake for a little while, because we *just* floated down the Fortymile and got to the Yukon. It became apparent after a little bit of paddling that getting that dredge into the middle of the canoe was a mistake, because the person in the front was super light and there was me in the back—and then this damn dredge in the middle. Well it turns out we discovered we couldn't aim; we couldn't control the boat.

This weight—it probably weighed 150 lbs—was just too much for us to overcome. So here we were drifting out, heading more towards the center of the Yukon. And let me tell you, that was foreboding. The Yukon flows at about 7 miles an hour and the current is strong enough that you can't seem to manage to do anything. Well we were slowly moving across the river. And that's exactly what we didn't want to do, because we didn't want to end up on the far bank. Then we would have to somehow get back. Getting rid of that dredge probably would have helped considerably.

So anyway we're going along here trying different things and pretty soon we discovered we could back paddle and go backwards and head towards the shore we wanted to be on. So we did that until we finally got over to the shore and celebrated with a "whoopee" or two. Then we hooked the line on the boat and just lined it down the river so we would have control.[28]

---

28    Cecil Kuhne, *Canoeing*, Mechanicsburg: Stackpole Books, April 1,1998, 94–95. Tim and his friend used the rope to guide the boat down the river as they walked down the shore. This "lining" method is often used to safely get a boat down rapids or dangerous waters—if, of course, the shoreline allows you to walk along it. The process has its own dangers if the boat travels faster than the walker (turning the walker into a swimmer) among other things.

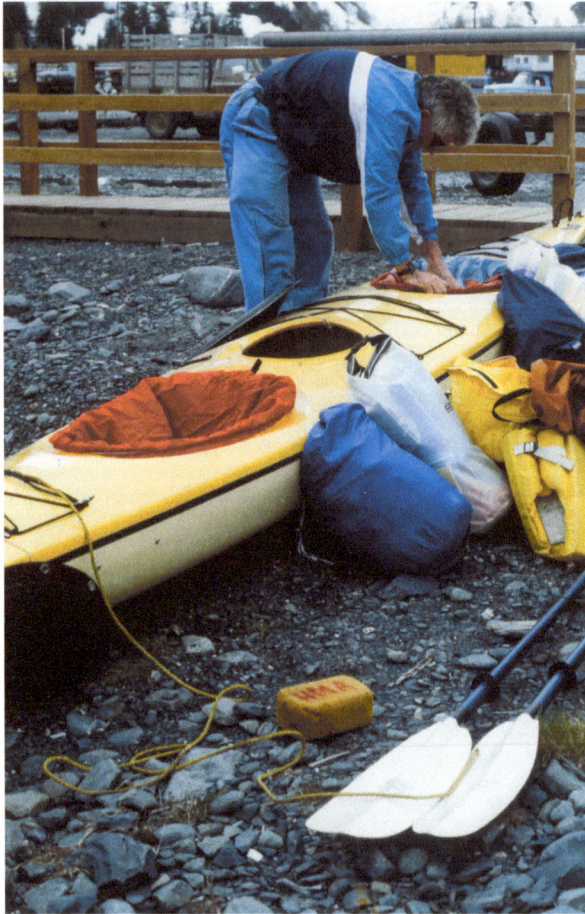

*Preparing for Blackstone Bay (Prince William Sound)*

Photo by Bonnie L. Campbell

## Bear

Well most stories that center around doing something out of doors on a trail or a road or something ends up being a bear story. And if you don't have one people always ask you "Did you see a bear? Did you have a bear problem?" This story has a story about a bear and that is when Bonnie and I went on a kayak trip in Prince William Sound out of Whittier. We rented a kayak and scooted off to the end of the bay and decided we were going to camp down here at the end of the bay.

The shore there is very rocky and kind of has ripples from storm action that through the years accumulate piles of gravel—kind of rolls.

Some of them are maybe three-, four-feet-high. So we decided to camp, to find a nice spot and camp. So I told Bonnie just sit tight and keep the boat pointed in with the paddles and I'll go up and take a look and see if there's a flat spot. As I was walking up the trail, I think I heard Bonnie yell, or something caught my attention. I looked up and realized there was a bear not running but walking towards me, probably not more than 20 or 30 feet away by the time I saw it. It was coming over one of these ripples of gravel. So I did the prudent thing—I turned around and took off running as fast as I could, told her to "push off". And she did. We got out of there finally and ultimately went down on some other spot on another beach.

But when I got back in the kayak, Bonnie was laughing and just couldn't hold herself *back*. She thought that was *so* funny. She said you can't believe how funny the two of you looked. What happened is the bear took off in one direction and I took off in the other. Bonnie was sitting in the kayak just laughing away.

That wasn't a dramatic bear story, but it was a bear and there was nothing really dangerous about what happened. If you spend much time in Alaska, you'll end up with an encounter or two with a bear, and most of them end up on the good side.

## Stuckagain

Well I was just looking at some of the stuff we'd written about and what not. I realized there was one little piece of excitement one time that I managed to do. And that had to do with a bear. I'd ridden my bike up Stuckagain Heights Road and was turned around getting ready to head down. For people who have—*or haven't*—been on Stuckagain Heights Road there are a couple little dips that slow you down slightly once you start. Once you get cooking you can get hit 30, maybe 40 miles an hour. Well, I got to the point I was hitting probably 30 miles an hour.

I was just past the last house on Stuckagain Heights Road going downhill. All of a sudden I just see this blur—it was a bear. It came from the left side of the road and it wanted to cross to the right and ran right in front of me. I didn't have any time to get on the breaks at all. So actually what did happen, it's hard to believe, but I hit the bear on my bike—but I didn't fall over—I stayed upright. And I had my face in the bear fur. I could smell it. I decided I'd better get out of here. I could hear scratching — like claws on the asphalt—and I figured probably I scared the bear probably as bad as it scared me. But in case that wasn't the case, I wasn't going to spend any time looking around. I started pedaling as fast as I could to make sure I put some distance between me and that bear.

## Beach Ball in the Sky

A few years ago a friend of mine and I decided it was such a beautiful week or two of weather and still cold and good skiing. We decided to fly into the Ruth Glacier to do some skiing, climbing, and Telemark skiing—just kind of enjoy good snow and good daylight. It was probably about April. Temperatures were real reasonable.

So we flew in with one of the glacier pilots and set up camp on a beautiful little knoll. *We* proceeded to ski around there a couple days. We dug out a kitchen so that if it got windy we could have a place to get down, be able to cook, and be in shelter without having to put the stove in the tent and put it at risk of burning up. Anyway I was in the hole—in the snow a couple feet deep. Then I thought I heard some noise. Well there were only the two of us out there on this glacier. And there was nobody for miles. So I thought something must be up. So I got out and see this woman was pretty excited and she said "Did you see that? Did you see that?"

And I said "See what?"

She said "That thing in the sky up there?"

I said "I didn't see anything. What, what did you see?"

She was in the process of trying to explain it to me, what she saw when all of a sudden off the horizon *I saw* this ball. It looked like an orange ball of something. Perfectly round like a big beach ball. We stood there and just stared at it, trying to figure out what on earth it could possibly be. Then this thing, this big ball, developed *something* like a hole in the bottom. It was like *some* liquid came pouring out and eventually *it* just dissipated and disappeared.

Of course we were further away from this thing than we could reasonably get to, to see if there was anything there. And we were reluctant to go. Especially since we had no idea what it was what was going on. We had no idea. So that night we went to sleep in the tent. Not really a restful night, but thinking what on earth could that possibly have been?

And you know, just in a matter of minutes after this thing started to appear to leak, it disappeared. So there was nothing we could do. Just looking around was the only thing we could do, and there was nobody around. But we knew that the pilot was coming back in to bring another couple skiers in later on. And as soon as he got there we skied down to the plane and asked him "Geez, did you see the strange light in the sky last night?"

And he laughs and he says "Yeah, yeah. Everybody's talking about it."

I said "What do you mean, everybody's talking about it?"

"Well, it was an experiment that the University of Alaska did up on their missile range out at Poker Flats or whatever it is. And what they did is they shot a barium ball into the sky which would illuminate and then just disappear like it did. But what they were trying to do is to see if they could activate the northern lights, artificially."

Well, we knew that it wasn't the northern lights, because we'd been in Alaska long enough to see the northern lights several times and this was <u>not</u> the northern lights. This was a big ball. Anyway, so that explained it. He said that the University of Alaska, Fairbanks did it, but they forgot to notify the news media about this event happening. And so it precipitated a lot of people calling in thinking they were seeing some spaceship or something. So that mystery was soon solved and we had a good laugh about that and went on about our business.

## UFO

Well everybody has to have an unidentified flying object type of experience. And mine happened one night when I was working in Valdez and drove back from Valdez back to Anchorage about ten o'clock at night. It was about two days before Christmas. There was nobody on the highway. Nobody.

So I'm driving down the highway and I look up at my windshield and—what's this? It looked like a reflection of some lights going across the upper part of my windshield. Like Christmas tree lights. They looked like they were being towed by something. And there's nothing out there. There's no body. There's nobody for miles around out there.

In Vietnam we had C-130 airplanes that had machine guns mounted on the side of the plane. When they had some enemy action that they wanted to get rid of, they'd bring in one of these planes; fly slowly over and open fire with the machine guns, rocket launchers, and everything else they can think of. We called them "Puff the Magic Dragon." And I only saw them operate a couple of times. But that was what I thought about when I saw these lights in the sky.

So anyway I stopped my car and got out. And then I noticed there was a car coming up behind me. It was the only car I'd seen since I left Valdez. And the car pulled up behind mine and stopped, this lady got out. She said something to the effect "Did you see those lights?"

I said "Sure did. Did you see 'em?"

She said "Yes."

And I said "That's two of us." So we weren't seeing things. There must have been some kind of lights up there. So we talked about it and then they disappeared. These lights were kind of coming straight at me, but very high. They were higher than the ridge of the mountains—I was in kind of a semi-valley. These lights were above that. Then they made kind of like a right turn and went off another direction, then just disappeared. But they were visible for couple minutes at least, it's hard to say.

*The lady* said she was going to go up to one of the pipeline pump stations, which was about ten miles from where we were, *to* see if anybody has seen these lights. I think she gave me her phone number or something. We were going to call and see if anything turned up in the news in the morning. I continued on home. Actually I got up to Glennallen, went in the all night quick stop and there were two guys there. I asked "Did any of you guys see some lights here a while back in the sky?"

And the one guy said "No, didn't see anything."

And the other guy said "Yeah." He said "They looked like Christmas lights?"

I said "Yeah."

He's seen them. Anyway, I continued on home. The next morning I got up and called the radio station I normally listened to and asked them if they had any reports of these lights. And they said yeah, they did. They said it was reported by a northwest airlines pilot coming into Anchorage from the lower 48 someplace. And the pilot said that he encountered in the distance from him, some lights that were like Christmas lights — multicolored, like a string of lights, only a big wad of them.

So they put it on the news that a northwest airlines pilot had seen these lights and described what he had seen. I called up the radio station again later on. They told me, "Well, the official word is 'nobody has seen anything.'" You had to be imagining that. The authorities say there was nothing there." No lights, and we were all kind of imagining things.

Well, I'm sure with that approach nobody's going to investigate it or report anything else about it. But it was interesting. And who knows. I certainly don't at this point in my life.

# REFLECTIONS

# THINKING ON IT

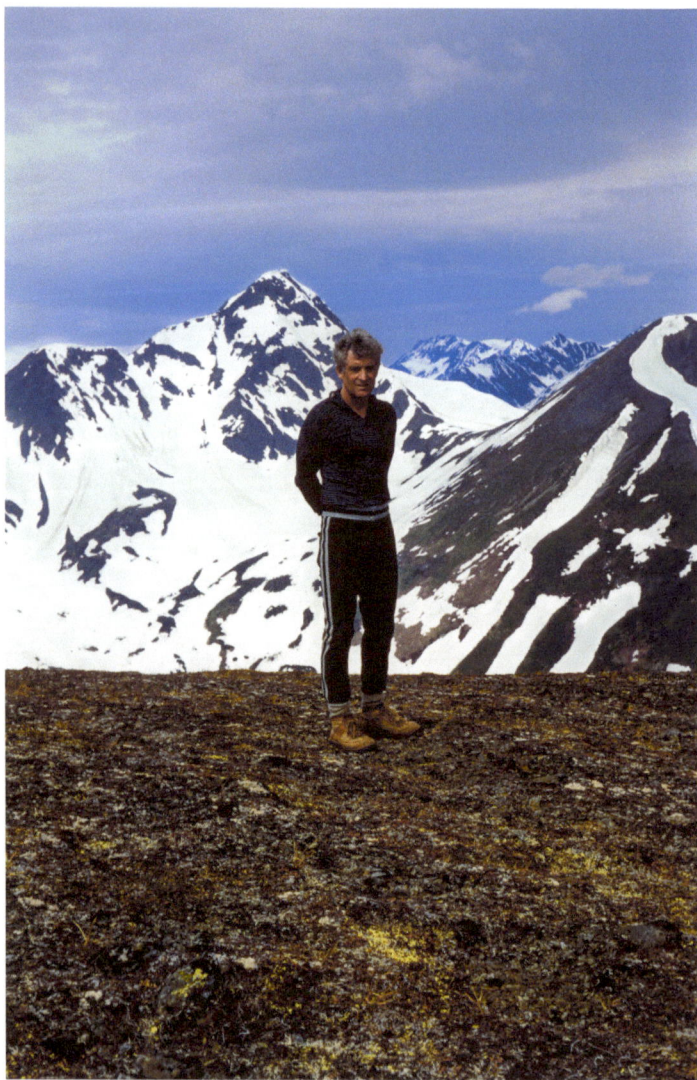

*Hiking in the Chugach*

Photo by Bonnie L. Campbell

## Lists

A t some point I thought I would like to list all the different things that I have done and make sure that I share with other people some of these activities I've done.

## Hardest Job

Like what is the hardest job that I ever done that I actually made a living at? Such as the one time I worked making laminated wood beams, which was probably one of the most physical jobs I ever had.

It was pounding wood—2x4s, 4x4s, 4x at various lengths. Twelve feet. Twenty feet. And you had these were glue lams, and you put glue on both sides of these different sized wood and then you start pounding on it with a big, huge mallet that probably weighed sixty pounds. And you pounded the wood so that they were even. And you just beat on this wood. Even moving them a quarter of an inch was a big deal. And after you pounded them, got them as close as possible; then you ran them through a mill and cut them to size. But you had to take these—it's really hard to describe. Especially when you don't know what the hell you are talking about, but it was just a very strenuous job.

*It was the* kind of a job that after work nothing tasted better than a good cold beer. Especially in a really hot day and especially *since* we were building these laminated wood beams in this big old building. During the day it would get hot. Anyway, this had to be one of the hardest jobs I ever had. I think we got paid two dollars an hour. Can't believe we got paid so little for so much work, but that's the way it went.

## Best Places

*Next I'd like to list* some of the best places I've been and *things I've* done.

One of the most fun things I ever did was when Ellyn Brown and I did the Rogaine race. I guess you'd call it a race, up by Trapper Creek. There's that whole article that Ellyn had written up that's included here. Ellyn did a tremendous job writing it up. But I think we both agree, and I think most of the people that did the event agree that it was really a lot of fun. And talk about a job. Bill Spencer and Dan Ellsworth did an amazing job on setting this course up and making it run right, because it was a twenty-four hour type of a thing, covered twenty-seven or thirty, I can't remember—a lot of miles. But anyway the story is included in my story here.

One other event that I participated in that was pretty outstanding was the world senior games at St. George, Utah. They were bike races, they had mountain bike and road bike races — four of each. But since I was flying my bike around, I just did road bike races. They had a first class outfit from San Diego that would set up the timing, set up the races, set up the results. And did it all somewhat you might say computerized. But it was really fun to do a race that was so well organized and really just a lot of fun. Plus St. George, Utah is a nice place to ride your bike.

Living with Parkinson's

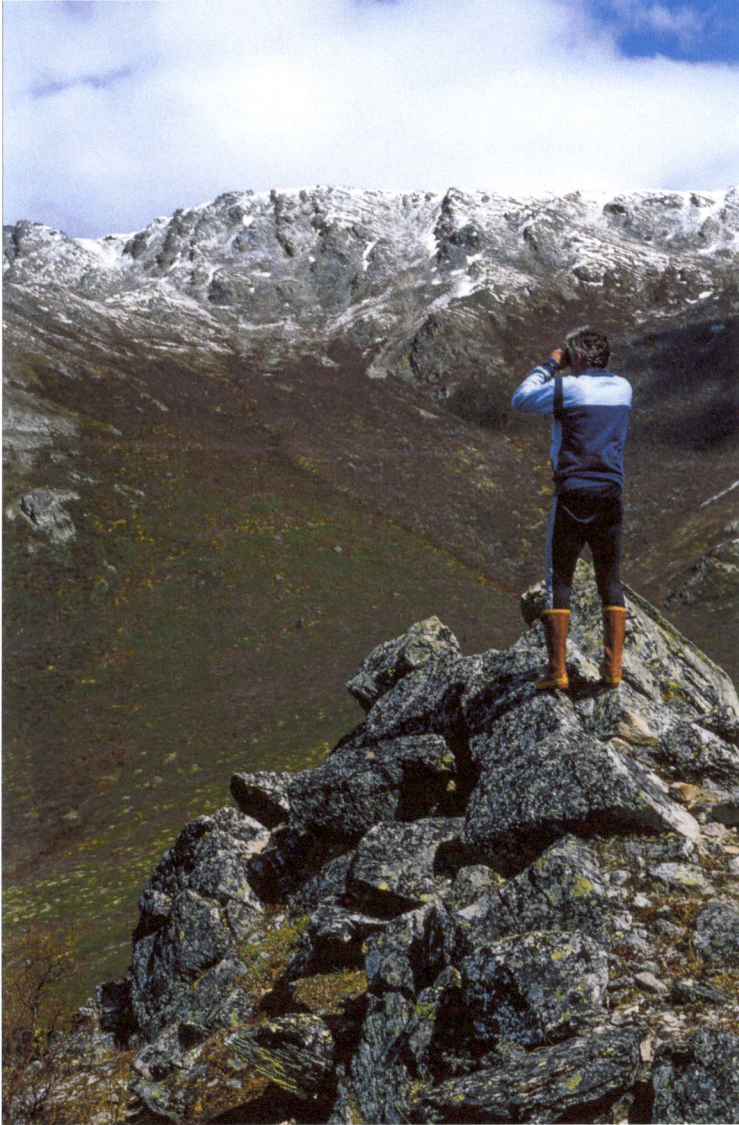

*Searching for Rams, Denali National Park*

Photo by Bonnie L. Campbell

*Not long ago, Tim agreed to help with a series prepared by Anchorage KTVA television reporter Lauren Maxwell called "Caring for Your Parents: Coping with Dementia." At that time, Tim continued to work out at the gym. He even walked home at times, though it was always a possibility that he'd have to ask how to get there. The message it seemed—life is meant to be lived—even when there are significant challenges.*

*Parkinson's disease and Lewy body dementia continue to impact his body and his memory—particularly short term memory. Imagine trying to articulate things that are important to you, yet continually losing your train of thought. Or trying to find your train of thought only to realize it left the station and you aren't quite sure which track to follow.*

Now as I draw to a close on this and I think back on it—What did I forget? Who did I forget? And all that. Well the answer to that is simple. I don't forget, but I don't remember all these different people that through the years have helped me and got me into things like orienteering, running, running races, bikes, bike races, skiing, skiing and ski races.

I still think that one of the most fun of my activities that I had the pleasure of doing was with Ellyn Brown was when we did the first Rogaine. Up at Trapper Creek, no… Where was it? I don't know. It was up out of Trapper Creek wherever that is. But anyway. To start off with that took a monumental effort for Bill and Dan Ellsworth to put the whole thing together and make it to come out as smooth and as fun as it was. I would hope that this could be replicated. Unfortunately it's not going to be me. I'm now behind the eight ball, and probably will stay there the rest of my life.

Which just brings me to a conclusion is that I've had a good run in life and enjoyed it. Met some great people. Did some great activities. I could start naming them off, but. Write down St. George, Utah, hiking in Death Valley for a couple of weeks. Some of these things are just genuinely fun. But I can't remember. Some of them are just leaving my memory. So I wanted to get this done before I had significant loss to my memory. But that's a battle that all of us will face eventually. At least I've been told that. I think sometimes from this ungodly number of little pink pills, white pills, green pills, orange peels that some of this has helped, will help me—I'm not sure what. Get along better in the last few years of my life? Whatever that is? Or just make me kind of a, a vegetable? Nobody wants to do that.

So again, the number of people I could name would be insurmountable. And I wouldn't want to try to do it because invariably I'd leave somebody out that was a significant player in part of my life. We kind of go in and out of each other's lives.

When I was in the military and getting out of the military. I was stationed *at* Fort Ord, California and I got into Experimentation Command — whatever that is. But it was actually a group and our job was to do an experiment. And since all this stuff is obsolete, I don't think it's classified. Just in case, we'll play on the safe side. — All that did was make me forget more. — Like what was I going to say, and why didn't I say it when I knew it and not now? Two minutes later when I don't know it?

My only suggestion in life here for anybody who wants a suggestion, and probably doesn't, but I'll give it to them anyway. That is, prepare yourself for the future. Because you may end up living out there for a long time. And the more comfortably you can live, probably the happier you'll be. We can't predict how long we'll live obviously, but all of us here probably are good for another few years. So being prepared, like having the ability to select some kind of an old folks or a caregivers home. I know I didn't.

I didn't really think about it too much until I would come home from working or doing something and I discovered I couldn't remember things. And I mean significant things. Like I couldn't remember what I did earlier that day. But my long term memory is, I won't say it's pretty much intact, but it's pretty good. You know, I can pull things out of it. It's like I say, if you want to record that or keep that information for your children or people who may be interested, then start on it at least sooner than later. Because later *is going to* be never. And that's just going to turn into a rambling exercise of what the hell ever happened to my memory?

I mentioned it a couple different times, in a couple different places, but there are things that I have done, things that probably I will do the rest of my life, and things that I definitely won't do for the rest of my life. And I'm very sad about *that*, but that's... that's just the way it is. Like Mount Marathon. I'll never run Mount Marathon again.[29] That doesn't mean that at some point that I can't enjoy it. Just that right now it's a little awkward, but that's okay.

I've thought about naming, thanking all the people that have done things for me. Or that have affected me directly and indirectly. But I started making a list a couple times and what they do. And I decided that that would be a big task and I'm afraid that I could botch that one up and that I could forget a lot of names. But there are people who are special.

Ellyn Brown is great person and doing great things athletically and is the kind of a person that you or anybody else would want to be around because she's upbeat. She was upbeat with me when I discovered that I probably had Parkinson's disease. And that that was a real downer. And by the time I got into a doctor that dealt with Parkinson's and Alzheimer's diseases, I realized that it's not something that a Band-Aid or an aspirin pill will in any way take care of.

So here we are in life. This disease, Parkinson's with Lewy Body dementia. I think it's probably not a good thing. And I think that I'm not going to be the last one to get it. So, hopefully there will be some research done that may or may not cause some positive thing along with Parkinson or Alzheimer's. They're not very happy diseases. They're kind of crude little devices, because it limits what you can do. Like you can't run or I mean I can't. Maybe people with Parkinson's can get around this, but I can't run, I can't ride my bike. I can't jump. I can't do Mount Marathon. I can't do a lot of these things that I used to do and didn't think much about them. But once you have the disease, then you have to deal with it. Unfortunately. And there's a bunch of statistics and information on it, but I'm not going to try to pull all that information up out of the computer which I can't operate anyway, and make it a part

---

29    Seward Chamber of Commerce, "Mount Marathon Longevity Awards." *Seward.com* accessed December 20, 2013, http://mmr.seward.com/results/longevity-awards/. For many Alaskan mountain runners the Seward Mount Marathon race on July 4th is an annual highlight. In 2009 Tim received a longevity award for racing Mount Marathon 30 times. As of 2013, only eight men have completed the race that many times or more.

of this rambling little story. My only suggestion is that people take the time to inform themselves about these diseases and what they can do about it because there is some news on that front. My friend Barbara can ferret out that information better than I or anybody I know can.

Finally the list of things that I've done and going to do and thought I could do. Some of them I did, some of them I didn't. But those that I did I was very fortunate that I had enough time in life to be able to do. My bicycle around Tasmania and other parts of Australia—I think everybody knows that what has caused me to look at my life again, because I have got a bad case of Parkinson's disease. And the doctors tell me that it's not something that's curable. And you have it and you'll have it the rest of your life. So live with it. But in this process I've discovered that Parkinson's and Lewy Body dementia are very limiting in what I can and cannot do. Such as go for a run, go for a bike ride. I could do a lot of those things, but it's a forever. If I go for a two mile bike ride is a big deal. I hope that something good comes out of the research that scientists and people are looking at. Like Parkinson's and Lewy Body dementia, and any other disease. Of course those I'm particularly interested in.

### Thank You

I want to thank everybody that helped me on this book and just, not only my book, but I do genuinely, sincerely want to thank all those people that have helped me through these last few years and made my life somewhat palatable. I thought about mentioning names. There would be so many people that I could thank and would want to thank. Except that, I feel I can't do justice to it, because just sure as hell I'd miss a name or two of some people that were very significant and my memory being what it's beginning to be I'd just space them out. But I wish I could list all these people somehow. Maybe at some point when I get wrapped up and my life has come back to some normalcy I might be able to do that. I might be able to thank people by name and for what they did.

Anyway, of course I want to thank this guy Jose who so dutifully transcribes everything and gets it into the right format.

*Jesse interjects: "I'm not Jose."*

Jesus.

*"The name is Jesse Tim."*

I've just been corrected. The name is Jesse.

And Bonnie. Bonnie has been masterful. If we ever do get anything like the likes of a book or magazine article or maybe nothing more than a little blurb in a magazine about some people that took it upon themselves to try to make a book about stories and about things that went on in a different time. I say that because the time that my parents lived, the time that I live, the time that my brothers live—it's all different and it's changing extremely rapidly. Fifteen years ago didn't even know what a computer was. Today Jesse has a cell phone that can probably do more things with that cell phone than I can with the best computer that I would have had at that time before I got sick. So anyway I think that I'll bring it to a close. Being as how I can't say enough about how these people have stepped up in the making the book, but also just in my life in general and how it's adjusted their life. Anyway. I think we'll close off at that point.

### Balance & Gratefulness

I think that the problem I have with this disease is that to date there's no upside. There's only downside. In other words, there's been no science to indicate that this disease has any kind of a point that would turn it around. It's a regressive disease, albeit slow. They say nobody dies of Parkinson's, but you just deteriorate. One of the things that I have disliked the most about Parkinson's is it keeps me from doing things that I've always wanted to do and always thought I would be able to do. Like hike in the hills—run, ride my bicycle, ski.

I've noticed that these activities have become exceedingly hard through the last couple years. And it's mainly a function of balance. A lot of these activities that I do and have done are based on your ability to have some degree of balance. And balance is what I don't have anymore. I stumble and stutter step and do all kinds of things. And have to be extremely cautious, because like the other day I tripped going out to the mailbox. Walking along on my front driveway that I've walked on hundreds of times, but I just—just tripped on it. But I don't know what else I can say about it. I don't like to think about it actually, but I guess as long as I continue to have good friends that are willing to put up with my stumbling, bumbling along when we go on a walk. A walk used to be three or four miles; now a walk is three or four hundred yards. But there are always people like Ralph that are more than willing to go with me.

So I guess it's time to put this thing to rest and just think positive things. And think that someday that sometime there may be a cure or something that reverses the negative side of this disease.

I want to thank everybody that's helped me on this. There's too numerous a number of people for me to try to mention all of them, because if I do that then I'm going to skip half of them. The other thing on this disease that I almost forgot, and I don't know how I could almost forget it, but it's the memory—the loss of memory. It's easy to just say something and 15 seconds later completely forget what it was I said. And I forget things long term, but short term memory is absolutely shot. It's almost comical. It's amazing how fast I can lose total memory of something I could have discussed with someone 15 seconds earlier. But again, that's a big huge part for me of the downside of this disease.

Again I want to thank everybody that's helped and put up with me these last couple of years. I just can't imagine there could be a better group of people than I've been fortunate to have become associated with. Even though it's partly because of this disease, but partly it's because these people are good people. They'd be good people anywhere. They're worth knowing and having as friends.

So I'll say so long and hopefully something changes some day for the good.

## Legacy

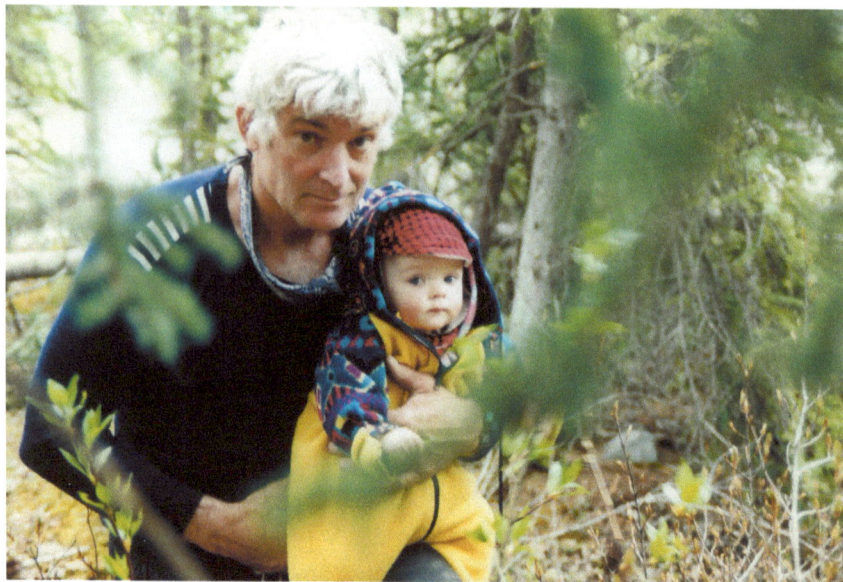

Photo by Shelly James

*Tim and Megan Hiking*

*Tim's daughter Megan is the light of his life. From Megan's school writing assignment below, it's clear he's shared his love of adventure.*

### Memories of a Child

Having an older father is very similar to living with a grandparent. He can be a nuisance, argumentative, and extremely forgetful, but will always accept me as myself and love me to the ends of the earth. As time passes, I get more and more scared. How much longer does he have? He is a man I will be ever grateful to for how he has affected my life. I hope my children will be able to know him as a grandfather to them.

My dad has always influenced my choices in life. He helped inspire my love of running, the joy of playing soccer, and the joy we both feel in biking and cross-country skiing. He is less of a parent and more of a loving grandfather, always wanting to spoil his little girl. In ways that is good because sometimes having one parent is definitely enough.

I remember when I was younger, and my dad would take me to a very fancy dress shop in the mall. I would always ogle at the gorgeous little frilly pink, blue and light green dresses. Their large satin bows shined in the shop light, and the lace would always ruffle quietly when someone walked by. Dad would tell me that they weren't for sale. He would tell me they were so special, like sculptures in a museum. I couldn't touch or have them. I accepted this, but we both would still go there, and look at the pretty dresses. In the store I would dance gracefully around pretending that I was dressed in one of those elegant gowns. Then I would always ask if we could go get a cheese roll from cars. And then we would usually head out to the airport to go get his mail.

For my 4th birthday that year my dad got me one of the pink fluffy dresses from the shop. It had a matching floppy silk hat. I never thought I would actually get to own a gown so extravagantly beautiful. He told me that because I was so special, I got to have their best dress. I wore it everywhere, even to the Tuesday Night Races. I felt like a princess, just like I imagined. When I twirled the skirt swirled around my little pink tights covering my legs. The silk on the inside was always cold and would give my skin goose bumps. I called it my party dress and wore it so much the seams started to tear. As I got older I moved away from this dress and passed it on to my younger friend. At this point in time I have no idea where it might be.

Now, of course, I know the store wasn't a museum. It moved or closed and I got older. My interests have changed from pink dresses and plastic high heel shoes to ski racing suits, and the newest carbon fiber road bike. Still, the time I enjoy will always be the same time spent with my dad. Not because he plunks his money down for anything that people say I look pretty in or will make me faster, but for the lessons he has taught me. The most important thing I think that he has taught me is to enjoy the little things in life and to use my imagination. Like in the dress shop, why buy one when you can imagine yourself wearing a different one anytime you wanted? My dad says, "Imagination is the key, and with it, you can unlock the door to a place that has and is what you want, need or desire." As I get older, my dad guides me into adventures that build my life story, and continues to teach me life lessons, I think half of them unintentionally. I will always value the imagination he helped grow in me, I feel it is the most important part of life. Even when he is gone these memories will still be with me, and with little effort I could recreate the adventures we had in our imaginations.

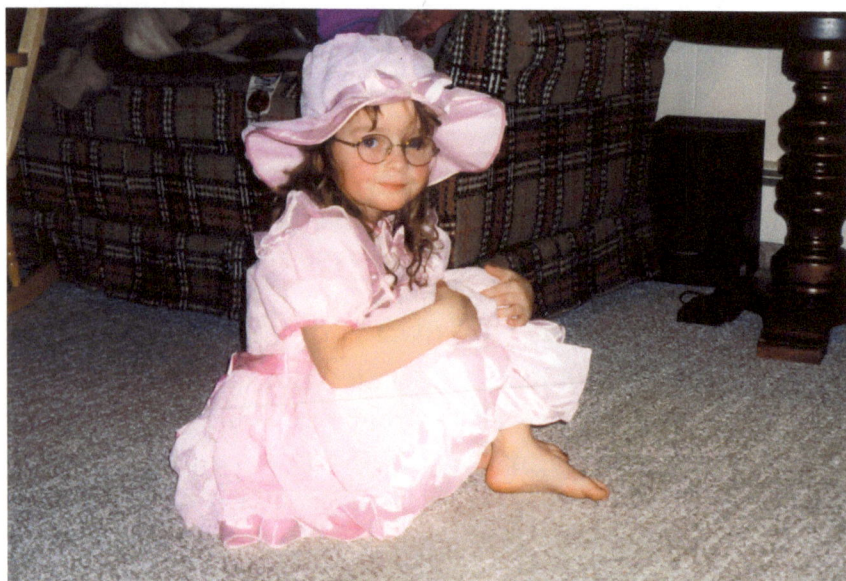

*Photo by Shelly James*

*Megan in the Pink Dress*

# REFERENCES

# BIBLIOGRAPHY

**Brown, Ellyn Gressit.** "Alaska Gold Strike Rogaine." *Orienteering North America*, July 1992, 21–22.

———. "Tangle Lakes Rogaine." *Orienteering North America*, November 1992, 12–13.

**Bureau of Land Management.** "BLM: Alaska: Homesteading Frequently Asked Questions." Bureau of Land Management, Department of the Interior. Accessed December 11, 2013. http://www.blm.gov/ak/st/en/prog/cultural/ak_history/homesteading/homesteading_Q_and_A.print.html.

**Cassidy, Jesse.** "The Story of 'Historical Badass' Ned Gillette | From Skiing Earth's Highest Summits to Being Shot to Death in Pakistan." *Snow Brains*, June 26, 2013. http://snowbrains.com/ned-gillette/.

**Carrs.** "Our Story." Safeway. Accessed December 16, 2013. http://www.carrsqc.com/ShopStores/Our-Story.page.

**David, E.J.R.** "Why it's time to (finally) officially rename Mount McKinley as Denali." *Alaska Dispatch*. February 12, 2013.

**Department of the Army.** "M-72 Series LAW, Operation and Function." Chap. 2 in *FM 3-23-25 (FM 23-25) Light Anti-Armor Weapons Field Manual*. Washington, DC: Department of the Army, August 30, 2001.

———. "'V' device." *Army Regulation 600–8–22 Military Awards*. 6-5. Washington, DC: Department of the Army, December 11, 2006.

**Frank, Michael.** "Historical Badass: Climber, Skier, Adventurer Ned Gillette." *Adventure Journal*, December 5, 2012. http://www.adventure-journal.com/2012/12/historical-badass-climber-skier-adventurer-ned-gillette/.

**Frommer, Arthur.** *Europe on 5 Dollars a Day.* New York: Arthur Frommer, 1957.

**Glines, C. V.** "William 'Billy' Mitchell: An Air Power Visionary." *Aviation History Magazine*, September 1997. Republished on Historynet.com, June 12, 2006. http://www.historynet.com/william-billy-mitchell-an-air-power-visionary.htm.

**Google.** "Blaine, WA to Dawson Creek, BC." *Google Maps.* Accessed June 26, 2013. https://maps.google.com.

**Govtrack.us.** "S. 155: A bill to designate a mountain in the State of Alaska as Denali." Accessed December 20, 2013. https://www.govtrack.us/congress/bills/113/s155.

**Komarnitsky, S. J.** "Mauling deaths mark 1st no-sighting of bear that killed runners," *Anchorage Daily News*, April 17th, 2007. http://web.archive.org/web/20070729112548/http://www.adn.com/bearattacks/story/204077.html.

**Kuhne, Cecil.** *Canoeing*, Mechanicsburg: Stackpole Books, April 1,1998, 94–95.

**Lewy Body Dementia Association.** "Home Page." Accessed December 16, 2013. http://www.lbda.org/.

**Manning, Harvey, ed.** *Mountaineering: Freedom of the Hills.* Seattle: The Mountaineers, 1960.

**Maxwell, Lauren.** "Caring for Your Parents Coping with Dementia." KTVA CBS 11 News. November 16, 2012. Anchorage, Alaska. http://web.archive.org/web/20130725142044/http://www.ktva.com/home/outbound-xml-feeds/Caring-for-Your-Parents-Coping-with-Dementia-179669401.html.

**McClinton, Blair.** "Summerfallow." In *Encyclopedia of Saskatchewan.* Regina: Canadian Plains Research Center, 2006. http://esask.uregina.ca/entry/summerfallow.html.

**Military Factory.** "M72 LAW (Light Anti-armor Weapon) Disposable Anti-tank Rocket Launcher (1963)." Accessed December 20, 2013. http://www.militaryfactory.com/smallarms/detail.asp?smallarms_id=72.

**Monsanto.** "Agent Orange: Background on Monsanto's Involvement." Accessed November 13, 2013. http://www.monsanto.com/newsviews/Pages/agent-orange-background-monsanto-involvement.aspx.

**Mountain Light.** "Mountain Light Press Release Monday, August 12, 2002." August 12, 2002. http://mountainlight.com/PR.html.

**National Geographic.** "Portuguese Man-of-War *Physalia physalis.*" Accessed November 24, 2013. http://animals.nationalgeographic.com/animals/invertebrates/portuguese-man-of-war/.

**National Park Service, Denali National Park and Preserve.** "Historical Timeline." Accessed December 11, 2013. http://www.nps.gov/dena/planyourvisit/climbinghistory.htm.

**National Transportation Safety Board.** "LAX02FA251." *NTSB Aviation Accident Database & Synopses.* Accessed June 26, 2013. http://www.ntsb.gov/aviationquery/brief2.aspx?ev_id=20020819X01425&ntsbno=LAX02FA251&akey=1.

**Neale, Megan.** "Memories of a Child". Unpublished school assignment.

**National Pesticide Information Center.** "DDT (General Fact Sheet)," Oregon State University. Corvallis: December 1999.

**Nordic Skiing Association of Anchorage.** "Trail History—Kincaid Park." Accessed December 16, 2013. http://www.anchoragenordicski.com/Trails/trailsKincaid.htm.

**Norris, Frank.** "New Highway Impacts and the Park Expansion Process, 1972–1980." Vol. 1, Chap. 8 in *Crown Jewel of the North: An Administrative History of Denali National Park and Preserve.* Anchorage: Alaska Regional Office National Park Service, U.S. Department of the Interior, 2006. http://www.nps.gov/dena/history-culture/upload/Vol%201,%20chapter%208.pdf.

**O'Flynn, Barry.** "The Sourdough Expedition to Mount McKinley" Irish Mountaineering Club, September 2007. http://www.irishmountaineeringclub.org/index.php?option=com_content&task=view&id=128&Itemid=89.

**Seward Chamber of Commerce.** "Mount Marathon Longevity Awards." Seward.com. Accessed December 20, 2013. http://mmr.seward.com/results/longevity-awards/.

**Twinlow Camping and Retreats.** "Camp Twinlow." Twinlow.org. Accessed June 26, 2013. http://twinlow.org.

**U.S. Senate Committee on Energy & Natural Resources.** "Sen. Murkowski Applauds Passage of Bill to Rename Mount McKinley." *Republican News.* U.S. Senate Commitee on Energy & Natural Resources. June 18, 2013. http://www.energy.senate.gov/public/index.cfm/2013/6/ sen-murkowski-applauds-passage-of-bill-to-rename-mount-mckinley.

**Wikipedia.** "Checkpoint Charlie." *Wikipedia, The Free Encyclopedia.* Accessed November 24, 2013. http://en.wikipedia.org/wiki/ Checkpoint_Charlie.

www.ingramcontent.com/pod-product-compliance
Lightning Source LLC
Chambersburg PA
CBHW041307020426
42333CB00001B/3